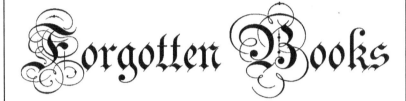
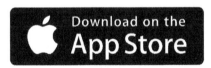
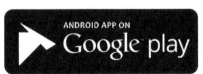

ISBN 978-1-332-26437-7
PIBN 10306242

1 MONTH OF FREE READING

at

www.ForgottenBooks.com

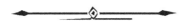

By purchasing this book you are eligible for one month membership to ForgottenBooks.com, giving you unlimited access to our entire collection of over 700,000 titles via our web site and mobile apps.

To claim your free month visit:

www.forgottenbooks.com/free306242

Similar Books Are Available from
www.forgottenbooks.com

HOW TO FEEL THE PULSE

AND WHAT TO FEEL IN IT

Works by the same Author.

Price 21s.

THE BRONCHI AND PULMONARY BLOOD-

VESSELS. Their Anatomy and Nomenclature; with
a criticism of Professor Aeby's views on the Bronchial
Tree of Mammalia and of Man. With 20 Illustrations.

J. & A. CHURCHILL, LONDON. 1889.

Price 5s. 6d.

CARDIAC OUTLINES FOR CLINICAL CLERKS

AND PRACTITIONERS; and first principles in the
Physical Examination of the Heart for the beginner.
With upwards of 60 Illustrations.

Intended as a Pocket Companion at the bedside. The
Outlines are designed to illustrate the methods and the
results of the examination of the heart in health and
in disease, and to assist the student in recording his
clinical observations.

A supply of Thoracic and Cardiac Outlines ($4\frac{1}{2}$ by $3\frac{3}{4}$
inches), on gummed paper, will be included in each
copy.

BAILLIÈRE, TINDALL & COX, LONDON. 1892.

[In the Press.

HOW TO FEEL THE PULSE

AND WHAT TO FEEL IN IT

PRACTICAL HINTS FOR BEGINNERS

BY

WILLIAM EWART, M.D. CANTAB., F.R.C.P.

PHYSICIAN TO ST. GEORGE'S HOSPITAL; CLINICAL LECTURER AND
TEACHER OF PRACTICAL MEDICINE IN THE MEDICAL SCHOOL; PHYSICIAN TO THE
BELGRAVE HOSPITAL FOR CHILDREN; ADDITIONAL EXAMINER IN 1891 FOR
THE 3RD M.B. OF THE UNIVERSITY OF CAMBRIDGE; LATE ASSISTANT
PHYSICIAN AND PATHOLOGIST TO THE BROMPTON HOSPITAL FOR
CONSUMPTION AND DISEASES OF THE CHEST

WITH TWELVE ILLUSTRATIONS

NEW YORK

WILLIAM WOOD & COMPANY

1892

TO

WILLIAM WADHAM

M.D., F.R.C.P.

CONSULTING PHYSICIAN TO ST. GEORGE'S HOSPITAL

AND FOR MANY YEARS

DEAN OF THE MEDICAL SCHOOL

AND

THE STUDENTS' FRIEND

THIS LITTLE BOOK FOR STUDENTS IS

GRATEFULLY INSCRIBED BY HIS CLINICAL PUPIL

THE AUTHOR

PREFACE.

THE old-fashioned art of feeling the pulse holds its own in medical practice, although very scant notice has been taken of it in modern medical literature. On the subject of the Sphygmograph, the student has at his disposal many and excellent books, and this volume would have had no purpose had it attempted to follow the same lines. It is specially devoted to matters which are scarcely touched upon in most books on the Pulse; but which are deemed of practical importance. It has been my aim to treat these in an elementary fashion, reserving for later publication merely theoretical or personal opinions. In spite of their imperfections these pages may perhaps be of service in directing the young student's attention to the oldest and not the least important of our methods of clinical study.

I am much indebted to the editor of Gray's Anatomy, Mr. T. Pickering Pick, and to the publishers, Messrs. Longmans and Green, for their leave to use two

plates from that work, and to Dr. Douglas Powell for
his kind permission to reproduce his valuable diagrams
of the pulse; also to my nephew, Mr. P. de Vaumas,
and to Dr. H. B. Grimsdale for their assistance in the
production of the other illustrations; and lastly, to my
friend Mr. Godfrey Thrupp for his valuable help in
revising the proofs.

WILLIAM EWART.

33 Curzon Street, Mayfair,
   March 1892.

TABLE OF CONTENTS.

CHAPTER I.

THE PULSE AND THE PRACTICAL METHODS FOR ITS STUDY.

TABLE OF CONTENTS.

CHAPTER II.

ELEMENTARY NOTIONS ON THE PHYSIOLOGY OF THE PULSE.

CHAPTER III.

THE CHIEF QUALITIES AND VARIETIES OF THE NORMAL PULSE.

CHAPTER IV.

THE CHIEF ABNORMALITIES OF THE PULSE.

CHAPTER V.

ON THE SIX CHIEF MORBID PULSE TYPES ; AND ON THE METHODS OF TESTING PULSES AS TO TENSION.

CHAPTER VI.

ASYNCHRONISM AND INEQUALITY OF THE PULSES.

CHAPTER VII.

CHAPTER VIII.

VENOUS PULSATION.

HOW TO FEEL THE PULSE
AND WHAT TO FEEL IN IT.

INTRODUCTORY.

THE vast importance of the various features of the pulse was guessed by physicians long before the discovery of the circulation, but it has only been fully demonstrated within the memory of living men. It would be unfair to suppose that all the labour which was devoted to the pulse by our early predecessors in their numerous treatises (Galen alone wrote seven) had been wasted and barren in practical results, but the amount of definite information to be extracted from them is remarkably small and buried in a mass of extravagant assumption. All empty surmises have now been cleared away, and the clinical uses of the pulse narrowed down to substantial facts connected with it, which might be recorded in a few pages. But the value of these clinical facts, few as they may be, is in advance of anything dreamt of before, and is the result of vastly improved anatomical and pathological knowledge. It is already capable of demonstration by the instrumental methods of physiology, and we are rapidly approaching a stage when some of the qualities of the pulse will find a mathematical expression.

A

Meanwhile, *the pulse has still to be felt.* But it is an operation of far greater importance to students of medicine nowadays than it was to those of long ago. Having much more definite objects in view in examining the pulse, we should not be inferior to them in the attention bestowed upon the examination. Moreover, since all experimental results are dependent upon the conditions of the experiment, we should take care that, even in apparently so trivial an operation as feeling the pulse, we use the best available method; in seeking for which we must be prepared to consider matters in some detail.

The following are the subjects dealt with in this book, and their order:

The matter having been arranged in short paragraphs with special headings, an index has not been deemed necessary; but a short glossary of the terms used formerly, and at the present time, has been appended.

CHAPTER I.

THE PULSE AND THE PRACTICAL METHODS FOR ITS STUDY.

———•◦•———

THE PULSE: CIRCUMSTANCES AND SITUATIONS FAVOURABLE FOR ITS DETECTION.

The Visible Pulse and the Tangible Pulse.

In common language " pulse " is synonymous with the pulsation at the wrist. But accuracy demands the prefix of " radial " to this particular pulse as there are various situations in which arterial pulsation can be seen as well as felt; while in others it can be felt, though not seen. When we speak of the pulsation being visible or palpable, we do not always mean that the pulse is easily seen or easily felt. Sometimes pulsation is quite obvious and even obtrusive, but, as a rule, we have to look very closely for any evidence of movement in the situations where the pulse is stated to be visible ; and in the same manner we must feel and feel again before we may safely say that we are unable to discover pulsation where pulsation should be felt.

Circumstances Favouring or Hindering the Detection of Arterial Pulsation.

No device *except position, a good light, and the use of a lens,* can help the eye in perceiving the pulsation of an artery if feeble. Palpation, on the other hand, is much assisted by a little knowledge and previous practice. Independently, moreover, of personal experi ence, there are definite conditions assisting, and others that hinder, success in the finger's search for the pulse. This is amply borne out by the experience of surgeons in various operations by which vessels are laid bare, and especially in those where an artery has to be found and tied. The operator, after exposing the vessel and whilst able to touch it, may be left in doubt as to its identity, or may even mistake it for some similar structure, "because unable to feel in it any pulsation." Yet, before the operation, the vessel may have been felt *to pulsate when pressed against bone or muscle.* Similarly, if the various arteries which are easily accessible to the touch be explored, it will be found that some pulsate much more distinctly and others less so; that those arteries which are supported by a firmer back-ground pulsate more powerfully than others; and, lastly, that pulsation is most strongly felt in those which are in proximity with bone. On the other hand, we shall become acquainted with arteries so superficially placed between thin skin and hard bone immediately underlying the skin, that the finger almost inevitably obliterates them in the attempt to feel their pulsation. Arteries thus situated do not afford very good opportunities for palpation, in spite of their superficial position. In conclusion, the *favourable conditions are:*

(1) *fair size of the artery;*
(2) *superficial course;*
(3) *a covering of thin skin;*
(4) *a supporting surface of muscle, cartilage, dense fascia, or bone* (note exception which follows).

The *unfavourable conditions* are : *the reverse* of the preceding ; and, in addition,—*immediate contact of an artery with underlying bone*, especially if the skin (as over the temple) be tightly stretched over the bone. Bony contact becomes then relatively a disadvantage.

I.

SITUATIONS IN WHICH PULSATION MAY BE SEEN IN LEAN SUBJECTS.

In the young, even when spare, and especially in children, the arterial pulses are *hardly ever visible*. At most, it may be possible to perceive the beat of the radial.

In old people, and especially in those of lean habit, several of the arteries will be seen to pulsate. This is due to the *atrophy of muscles* and of other tissues, or to the *senile dilatation and elongation* of the arteries, or to a combination of both.

The subjects of *aortic regurgitation* afford specially favourable opportunities, their pulsations being of exaggerated type, and their arteries large, whilst the patients themselves are generally thin.

Taking, then, the *most favourable subject,* a lean man, advanced in years, and suffering from aortic valvular incompetence, the following arteries would probably be seen to beat :—

The temporal artery.
The anterior and the posterior temporals.
The angular.
The facial.
Sometimes the transverse facial.
Sometimes the superior and inferior coronaries (at their origin).

The occipital (in cases of baldness).
The external carotid.
The common carotid.
Sometimes the subclavian.
Sometimes the innominate.
The long thoracic.
The axillary.
The brachial (especially near the bend of the elbow).
The radial.
The ulnar
The dorsalis indicis.
Sometimes the abdominal aorta.
The femoral (in the upper part of Scarpa's triangle).
Sometimes the inferior external articular.
Sometimes the malleolar branches.
Sometimes the anterior peroneal.
The dorsalis pedis.

In addition, pulsation may be seen in sundry small subcutaneous arteries, and, with the ophthalmoscope (*in cases of aortic reflux, of glaucoma, and sometimes in Graves' disease*) *in the retinal arteries.*

The Influence of Position.

In the case of several of the arteries enumerated above, the ease with which pulsation may be perceived *varies with the position of the patient or of the limb.* As special instances should be mentioned, *the radial* at the wrist, whose beat is favoured by very slight *flexion,* or at least by the *absence of extension;* the *ulnar,* whose pulsation may be visible in *slight extension* only; and especially the *brachial,* which becomes curved into a prominent loop above the fold of the elbow *when the limb is flexed.*

II.

SITUATIONS IN WHICH THE ARTERIAL PULSE MAY BE FELT IN MOST SUBJECTS.

With the exception of the smaller arteries, which are more easily seen than felt by the average observer, pulsation *is perceptible to the finger* in all arteries in which it is observed by the eye.

It is unnecessary to repeat here the list previously given, which applies to the special combination of senility and of emaciation with cardiac disease.

It was stated that during health, and in the young and sleek, the number of visibly pulsating arteries would be very small. This is not the case with the pulse as felt. In adults, even when presenting fairly thick integuments, the beat of the following arteries may usually be made out *on palpation :—*

The temporal artery.
The anterior and posterior temporals.
The occipital.
The facial.
The superior and inferior coronaries.
The external carotid.
The common carotid.
The subclavian.
The innominate.
The axillary.
The brachial (in its entire course).
The radial.
The ulnar (with difficulty).
Sometimes the princeps pollicis and the digitals (as a general pulsation of the pulp).
The abdominal aorta.

The external iliac.
The femoral (in the upper half the thigh).
The popliteal (in the lower part of the popliteal space).
The posterior tibial (at the ankle-joint).
Sometimes the anterior peroneal.
The anterior tibial (just above the ankle).
The dorsalis pedis
In special cases, the thyroids (as a general pulsation).

The Common Pulses.

Of this long series of arterial pulses *five only* are utilised in every-day medical practice :—
The temporal,
The facial,
The external carotid,
The brachial,
The radial.

III.

The Mode of Feeling the various Pulses.

The mode of feeling the radial pulse will be presently described at some length, and the best way of finding the other four will be thereafter briefly indicated.

Among the remaining pulses that of the *coronaries* may be felt *from the outside*, against the teeth as a background; but *better from the inside*, by grasping the thickness of the lip between two fingers.

The *innominate* and the *subclavian* beats will be felt by deeply plunging the finger into the *episternal notch* and into the *supra-clavicular fossa* respectively.

The beat of the subclavian is best felt where the

vessel lies on the surface of the *first rib*. That of the innominate is not readily, except in special cases, distinguishable from the strong impulse of the *arch of the aorta* communicated upwards.

In order to perceive *the axillary pulsation* the arm must be raised. The vessel can then be felt beating between the finger and the head of the humerus.

For the detection of *the external iliac* deep pressure must be made into the pelvis above Poupart's ligament.

Rather strong pressure is also required in the case of *the femoral*, if the thigh be muscular or very fat. The femur forms the background.

The popliteal pulse is more readily perceived when partial flexion has relaxed the tension of the powerful muscles among which the artery lies concealed.

The easiest way to feel the *posterior tibial beat* is to place the flat of the finger (whole length) in a vertical direction just behind the inner malleolus. *Soft pressure* of the phalanx against the os calcis will suffice.

The *dorsalis pedis* is readily felt pulsating when the finger is applied across the upper part of the arch of the foot. Here again the pressure should be soft, and the flat of the finger should be used.

IV.

The Seats of Election for a Study of the Pulse. The Radial Artery; its Advantages.

In most of the situations enumerated above, although the pulse may be recognised, it lies too deep to be successfully studied. For this purpose the seats of election are *the face* for the temporal and the facial arteries, *the arm* for the brachial, and *the wrist* for the radial. The first two vessels are almost too super-ficial. The radial, besides being much larger, possesses great advantages over them ; and over the brachial, it has that of personal convenience.

(1) *The radial* presents to perfection those ana-tomical conditions which were described on page p. 4 as rendering pulsation easy to feel. It is *superficial*, and it is backed by a *bony plane*. But it is not in imme-diate contact with bone at that part where the pulse is felt; although, nearer the wrist-joint, it lies on the styloid process, in close contact with its surface.

(2) Another great advantage of the radial is the *considerable length* (quite three inches) over which it is accessible to the touch. This enables the observer to feel the pulse *with three or even four fingers*.

DESCRIPTION OF THE PRACTICAL METHODS FOR THE STUDY OF THE PULSE.

I.

THE METHOD OF COUNTING THE PULSE.

The pulsating artery having been found, the next thing (because the easiest) is to count its beat. This is quite distinct from the operation of "feeling the pulse," which is an active and rather difficult inquiry Here the touch is almost entirely passive. The points requiring attention are :—

(1) To *keep touch with the pulse* by a gentle pressure, so that none of the beats are lost to the finger ;

FIG. I.

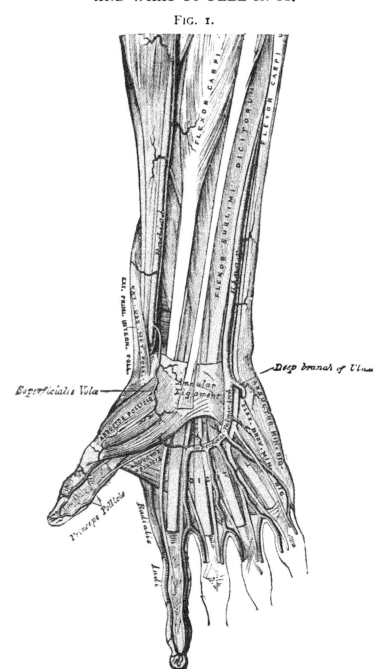

The Radial and Ulnar Arteries at the Wrist and the Superficial
Palmar Arch.

(*From Gray's "Anatomy," by permission.*)

(2) To *moderate the pressure* of the finger, so that none of the beats are suppressed by it ;

(3) To *avoid mistaking the pulse-beat of the finger* for that of the patient's radial artery. It is chiefly owing to the reality of this source of confusion that counting the pulse with the thumb has been condemned by authors; the beat of the *princeps pollicis* arteries being larger than that of the digitals, and rather more liable to be felt during the operation.

Various Sites for Counting the Pulse.

For a simple determination of the pulse-rate we are not limited to the radial artery ; *any artery will serve* which, being superficial, is of sufficient size to enable us to securely feel the beat. An opportunity often occurs of counting the pulse without awaking a *sleeping patient*, by lightly feeling the temporal artery where it crosses the zygomatic process. This method is especially useful in children. It is indispensable in cases of great restlessness and of delirium, and in chorea, where the arms are violently thrown about. It is also indispensable to the anæsthetist.

Counting the Pulse at the Carotid and at the Heart.

In the foregoing remarks it has been assumed that each systolic wave reached the periphery; but in exhaustion and in cardiac disease this is not always the case, and our observation must be a direct one—viz., by palpation or auscultation of the apex beat, after the method used in cases of apparent death for determining whether life is or is not extinct. Whenever the pulse has been taken *at the heart*, let the fact be noted.

It may sometimes be convenient to take the pulse of the *carotid artery* (see p. 33) if the wrists are not available or their pulse too weak, but especially during auscultation of the heart, when the first sound has to be timed from an artery as little distant from the heart as possible. In some diseases this beat is so prominent that the pulse may be counted *by sight* and without touching the patient. The same facility is also presented by the heart itself when the apex-beat is visible.

Duration of the Observation.

Although the *clinical unit of time is the minute*, our observations are, in practice, limited to fractions of a minute. Hence the necessity for a *watch beating the second*. A pulse beating regularly may be safely " taken " in fifteen seconds, less accurately in ten. An irregular, and especially an intermittent pulse, requires an observation lasting at least thirty seconds. In cases of unusual slowness or rapidity, it is well to make two separate observations of half a minute each, and to take the mean. The frequency of any intermissions, linked beats, or small beats, should be ascertained by separate observations.

Preliminary Precautions.

Since the pulse-rate varies with movement, change of posture, emotion, thought, and speech, it is well that the patient should be *at rest, supine, silent, and unexcited.* If sitting or standing, or if asleep, the fact should be noted. It will often save time to count the pulse before the patient has moved or spoken; but with some, who are nervous, the physician's approach is enough to cause excitement, and with them a later count would probably be more reliable.

Where the pulse is very rapid, weak, or irregular, considerable delicacy of touch—*i.e.*, considerable attention—may be required for its detection.

Rules to be followed in Counting the Pulse.

Rule I.—*Determine the number of beats in fifteen seconds, and, multiplying that by four, record the rate per minute.*

Rule II.—*If the pulse should be irregular in rhythm, count for thirty seconds, or else for two separate periods of fifteen seconds.*

Rule III.—*If the pulse should be very small or very slow, or faltering, count at the heart and record the fact. It is useful in these cases to record also the rate found at the wrist.*

Rule IV.—*Whenever possible, let the patient be reclining. If not in bed, let him be seated.*

Rule V.—*The patient should be silent and still, and judgment must be used in selecting a moment when no excitement prevails.*

II.

THE METHOD OF "FEELING THE PULSE."

I. GENERAL RULES RELATING TO THE ATTITUDE OF BODY AND LIMB.

The operation of "feeling" or "trying" the pulse *must always be kept separate* from the operation of "taking" the pulse. It claims the whole mind. Simple and purely mechanical in appearance, it is a combined effort of some of the higher functions, and requires skill in manipulation, keenness in observation, and other qualities which wait upon long practice and experience. Moreover, the data obtainable are meaningless apart from a knowledge of physiology and pathology.

That which has previously been said in this connection under the heading of counting the pulse applies here also, and need not be stated afresh. In all things success is largely dependent upon attention to small matters; and details such as the patient's attitude and that of the observer have their importance. The work of the draughtsman, of the musician, of the various artists and artisans is severally performed to greatest advantage in certain positions of the body, of the arm and of the hand. Of percussion the same is true and it is also true of feeling the pulse, where the touch has to be brought to bear with great delicacy. In most of the instances quoted movements of varying difficulties have to be performed. In this case it is the absence of movement that needs to be secured.

ATTITUDE OF THE BODY.

(1) The Observer's Attitude.

Attitude is of importance, because it facilitates, on the part of the observer, the appreciation of the pulse; and because in the case of the patient it influences the pulse itself.

For the observer almost any attitude may be made to answer so long as freedom from effort, and firmness are ensured. Certain things are nevertheless to be avoided. *Too great a distance* from the patient will necessitate stretching the arm : this is unfavourable. *Unsteadiness of muscle* will be greater in proportion to any fatigue;

—therefore if in the least tired the observer should be seated ; the body no longer needing to support itself, muscular work and reflex nervous work are thereby spared.

(2) The Patient's Attitude.

Many patients are aware that their pulse is influenced by position. *A fortiori* should the observer not lose sight of the *physiological variations*. It is normal for the pulse to become more powerful and rapid when the reclining posture is exchanged for the sitting or especially for the standing position; in feeble invalids, and even in nervous and weak persons, this difference may become considerable. Moreover, putting aside the direct influence thus exerted on the pulse, the patient's attitude may have some bearing on the success of the operation of feeling the pulse. In the case of *bedridden invalids* the *supine position* is the most natural and the best because the most supported. *When not bedridden*, it is desirable to cause the patient to *sit down* if previously standing. This will afford the student an opportunity of verifying for himself the accuracy of the statements made as regards variations of the pulse in changing position. Bearing all this in mind, it is well to establish for oneself a rule to take pulse observations on patients either in the supine or in the sitting position. If this practice should be occasionally departed from, a special note should be made of the fact.

ATTITUDE OF THE ARM.

Steadiness Essential ; how Secured.

Adequate support is essential for the observer's arm as well as for the patient's arm.

(1) *The observer's arm* is liable to oscillations arising from the heart's action. The less the support, so much the greater the instability from this cause. This is a first reason why the pulse should not be felt at arm's length. Again, for the same reason, accuracy of observation is out of the question under the influence of cardiac excitement from whatever cause; or during breathlessness induced by a rapid ascent. In practice the observer's arm most frequently seeks support on the bed, or on the table; but failing any mechanical support the upper arm should be gently steadied against the chest, allowing free play to the movements of the elbow and of the wrist.

(2) *The patient's arm*. Support in this case is yet more important, not only for the sake of steadiness, but because it often affords the simplest means for ensuring absolute relaxation of the muscles (see p. 19). The best plan, whenever manageable, is to cause the entire fore-arm and the hand to rest with their ulnar border *on bed or table*, the hand falling over in very slight pronation, so as to bear on the semiflexed joints of the 4th and 5th fingers.

Patient's Arm supported by the Observer.

Effectual support may be often afforded, according to another method, to the arm both of the patient and of the observer. The patient's left fore-arm is received on the observer's left hand and arm, so as to be supported almost in its entire length, whilst the observer's left elbow is steadied against the side of the chest. Again, when the pulse has to be felt under difficulties, for instance from a slight distance, or across the bed, as sometimes happens to the student in a crowded clinical class, the observer's grasp of the patient's wrist may both give and take a measure of support. In an attitude such as this the larger muscles come into play and much delicacy of touch cannot be expected. An observation taken under conditions so adverse cannot be a good one, though it may not be absolutely worthless.

MUSCULAR RELAXATION ESSENTIAL.

(1) In the Observer.

The first requisite for fine sensory appreciation is freedom from muscular strain. Any performance requiring skill is rendered difficult to beginners by misplaced energy. Their good intentions run into physical force. Yet of the latter very little is really needed. In this special case, as the words "feeling the pulse" imply, we are dealing with a sensory rather than a muscular function.

Adequate support may be said to be the cure for the muscular anxiety of all beginners. This is one of the chief reasons why any delicate work, be it of the hands as in fine dissection, or of the eye as in microscopic work, or of the ear as in auscultation, demands a firm basis. An excellent instance in point is afforded by the patient's strain, to which we shall presently refer.

(2) In the Patient—Management of the Patient's Wrist.

The chief difficulty arises in many cases from the *nimia diligentia* of the too willing patient. Complete muscular relaxation is needed: *first*, because muscular effort affects the pulse (a source of error which might be overlooked); *secondly*, because, under effort, the leaders will stand out at the wrist, placing the radial artery out of reach. Among hospital patients the student will recognise two types differing in the presence or in the absence of energy. The feeble and timid subjects usually allow the hand to lie on the bed; this is generally the case with female patients. Even they, however, if nervous, will involuntarily raise the wrist in opposition to our purpose, though they may allow the elbow to rest supported on the bed. On the other hand, the rough working man almost always presents his wrist, that is, raises his arm and stiffens his powerful muscles in moderate supination.

To such wrists the employment of any force is worse than useless; it will only aggravate the tension. The quickest method is to seemingly give up our attempt, to drop the stiffened arm, and to refuse it again if it be raised from the bed. When the patient has at last allowed the hand to remain at rest, the wrist is to be clasped with great gentleness by the observer's hand, whose fingers are then applied to the pulse. At the same time the thumb glides softly from the back of the radius to the back of the carpus, where a gradual and light pressure will almost at once succeed in *fully flexing the wrist*. This being effected, the spasm of the whole limb relaxes and the pulse is under control.

The Attitude of the Hand.

Before proceeding further we have two questions to consider :

(A) Which Pulse to hold?

As a constant rule that of the opposite side to that of the hand which feels. This is the only method which the learner can conveniently practise on himself. It may, however, be desirable to check the results of one position by those of the reverse one; and to feel the patient's left pulse with the left hand and his right pulse with the right hand, in addition to the previous experiment.

(B) Which Hand to Use?

It matters very little whether the right hand or the left hand be used.   There is obvious advantage in training both if possible.   Most observers however will fall into a one-sided habit, which probably will enable them to secure greater delicacy of touch at the expense of a little freedom.   This may have the advantage that the untrained hand can be brought to bear in cases of doubt, and, like the consultant's opinion, add new light through its comparative strangeness to the case.

The Attitude of the Observer's Hand.

Here, also, as far as the hand is concerned, the best position is depicted in the illustration.

As previously stated, the observer's right hand should hold the patient's left pulse and *vice versâ*.   It will be noticed that the *observer's thumb is applied to the back of the lower end of the radius:* this arches his wrist and raises the second phalanx from the patient's wrist.

A modification of the same method consists in *passing the thumb round the wrist* in such a manner that its extremity faces that of the fingers; or the thumb remaining unemployed over the back of the metacarpus, the ball of the thumb and of the little finger may be pressed against the back of the ulna.   In both these methods the hand encircles the wrist, and the last phalanx bears, not with its tip, but with its entire length, on the region of the radial beat.

FIG. 2.

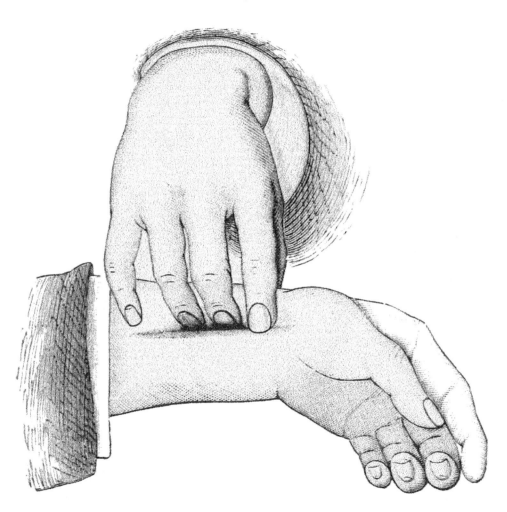

The " Superior " Position of hand to be adopted in feeling the pulse. In this illustration the index finger alone is shown in the act of *feeling*. The median and annular fingers are engaged in *compressing* the artery.

Although it is best to adopt the hand position first named, it is desirable for the . beginner to try every variety of position; and it is good at any time to test doubtful results by another method.

The "Superior" and the "Inferior" Position of the Hand.

When feeling his own pulse the student will observe that his finger tips may be made to approach it either

FIG. 3.

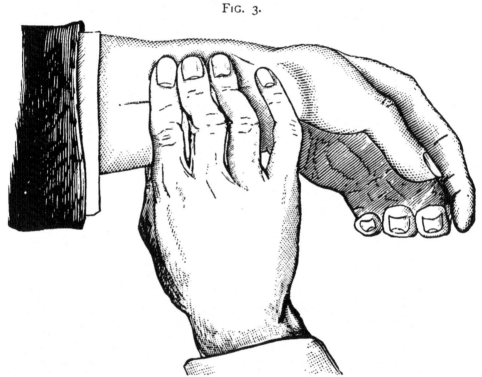

The "Inferior" Position of hand.—The right hand is, in this illustration, applied to the left wrist (as when the observer is taking *his own pulse*). If, however, the patient's *right pulse* be felt with the *right hand*, the index finger will then occupy the usual position, near the wrist. The fingers are shewn with the flat of the pulp applied to the artery, in the position most favourable for *feeling the pulse*.

with the palm of the hand turned upwards—or with the palm turned downwards. The position which has been described (see Fig. 2) represents the first of these two methods. I am in the habit of terming this the "*Superior,*" the other being the "*Inferior*" method (see Fig. 3). These names have reference to the relation of the fingers to the outer border of the radius.

The *superior position is the one to be adopted in all cases* by the student, except (for convenience) when trying his own pulse.

The Arrangement of the Fingers, and their Relation to the Wrist.

The simplest case, in which *one finger only* is applied to the pulse, requires no special description. Most observers prefer to use *two or even three fingers.* It is to this case that our remarks specially apply.

The Distal Position and the Proximal Position of the Index Finger.

(1) If we imagine that the observer's right hand is feeling the patient's left radial pulse from above, whilst his thumb rests on the back of the wrist, the employed fingers will be arranged in the following order:—*The index nearest the patient's hand; the median, in an intermediate position; the annular nearest the heart.* The same arrangement will prevail if the observer's left hand tries the patient's right pulse.

(2) If, on the contrary, the right pulse be felt from above by the observer's right hand, the situation of the fingers will be reversed—viz., the index will be nearest the heart; and the annular, nearest the hand.

The second arrangement is preferred by some. But the first arrangement has the support of considerable antiquity and appears to be not less excellent. It is decidedly more convenient in controlling a stiff wrist. (see p. 19). Beyond this there is really no superiority, worth arguing here, of one over the other method. On the other hand, the advantage to be obtained from uniformity in the method will repay us for strictly adhering to one or the other plan.

Let it be understood that the foregoing refers exclusively to the "superior method," which alone is recommended to the beginner for reasons which need not be set forth at length.

The Exact Spot where the Finger should be Placed.

The *distal finger*, whichever it be, should be placed on the artery *immediately above the base of the styloid process* of the radius. The other two fingers (if three be used) would be arranged in loose contact with each other. For the special purpose of estimating tension it is desirable to separate the two centrally placed fingers by an interval from that more distally placed (see Fig. 2). To this arrangement reference will be made later on.

The Inclination of the Fingers.

The direction of the distal phalanges as they rest on the pulse claims a moment's attention. According as the hand and fingers are more or less arched above the wrist, the last phalanx of each finger will be more or less vertically applied to the long axis of the radius and of the artery. The absolutely perpendicular position (see Figs. 4, 5, 6) is not desirable unless it have for its object the occlusion of the artery by pressure. *For the purpose of fine feeling a slight inclination (obliquity) of the phalanx is desirable.* This brings a very sensitive portion of the pulp (not that nearest the nail) to bear on the artery, namely, that portion which generally meets the pulp of the thumb in the simple movement of opposition. This portion seems specially adapted for such tactile explorations as require to be combined with slight pressure; whereas at the extreme tip of the pulp there exists, it is true, yet greater delicacy of surface-touch, but one easily blunted by the slightest pressure.

II. The Exploration of the Pulse.

The fingers having been securely placed over the beating artery the exploration of the pulse begins. This consists

A. *of the application of a varying amount of pressure to the artery;*

B. *of a careful notice of the behaviour of the pulse under each degree of pressure,*

C. *of a manipulation (or "fingering") of the pulse.*

A. The Degrees of Pressure to be Applied.

The amount of pressure may of course be varied almost indefinitely; but there are three degrees which it is convenient to single out from the rest, namely,

1. *The lightest possible touch of the finger;*
2. *The medium pressure.*
3. *The obliterating pressure.*

These three varieties are shown in the accompanying illustrations (taken from Dr. Douglas Powell's diagram), which do not however depict the proper attitude of the fingers, but simply the effect of their pressure on the artery.

FIG. 4.

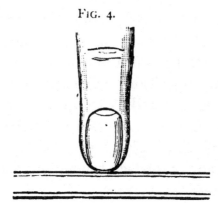

Shewing light pressure.

In Fig. 4 there *is bare contact* between the finger and the artery. The latter is felt, but is not compressed. *Very little pulsation is perceived.*

FIG. 5.

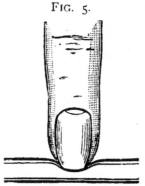

Shewing medium pressure.

In Fig. 5 the finger is applied with moderate force, and *the diameter* of the artery at that spot *is reduced by one-third, to one-half.* It is this degree of pressure which *yields the maximum sensation of arterial beat.*

FIG. 6

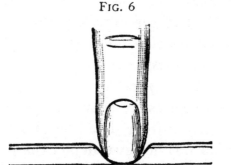

Shewing forcible pressure.

In Fig. 6 the finger bearing upon the artery *has flattened it.*

The deep pressure is made with the object of ascertaining the *amount of force,* or *the weight, which will completely abolish pulsation.* This is one of the most important parts of a systematic exploration of the pulse. The force required in order to extinguish the pulse will be found to *vary within very wide limits* in different individuals, and at different times.

We shall see later on that *a combination of deep and of medium pressure* is to be employed whenever we desire to ascertain that the obliterating pressure exerted by one or by two fingers has effected its purpose. In this case *the other finger is pressed moderately firmly at a point nearer the wrist,* in search of any vestige of pulsation, as shown in Fig. 2.

How to Regulate the Pressure.

Of the three degrees of pressure the third alone represents a definite result; it is a procedure requiring strength rather than skill. The other two degrees cannot be defined with precision (since they must vary with each individual strength of pulse), but must be left to personal judgment and experience. To those gifted with delicate touch, or trained to artistic pursuits, any suggestions are almost superfluous; but some beginners will find assistance in the following hints :

1. *On first applying the fingers exert rather firm pressure,* so as thoroughly to feel the beat;

2. *Almost immediately relax the pressure,* but let this be done *gradually* so that the finger is gently raised by the artery or would even seem to lift the artery with it;

3. *By degrees reduce the pressure to the utmost,* so that bare contact remains with the skin covering the

artery. *This is the first degree.* After observing the pulse at this stage,

4. *Proceed now to use active exploring pressure* and determine the amount which gives the maximum pulsation. *This is the second or medium degree;*

5. *Lastly gauge the resistance* of the pulse by using as much pressure as will obliterate the artery.

N.B.—*A quick and most practical way of gaining an idea of the procedure to be followed, consists in getting in succession two or three senior fellow-students to feel one's own pulse. The different sensations conveyed to the wrist by different observers will be more suggestive than the most elaborate descriptions.*

B. The Behaviour of the Pulse under Varying Pressures.

This is the tale which each artery under observation must tell for itself. The special points which have to be appreciated and described are indicated in Chapter II.

C. The Manipulation, or "Fingering," of the Pulse.

Hitherto the fingers have been stationary, and the presence or absence, the degree or quality, of the arterial beats have been their object of study. The present heading refers to a separate inquiry, in conducting which, *movements of the fingers must be combined with their tactile function.* It is no longer the pulse-beat alone, but also the artery itself, during the interval *between the beats,* or *whilst obliterated* by pressure, which comes under observation. Arteries differ greatly in their shape, size, and other qualities, as will be seen hereafter (see p. 58). Some of their changes being of much importance, we should avail ourselves of the information concerning them which may be gained by the two simple movements of the fingers about to be described

A gliding or rubbing movement across the axis of the artery.

A similar movement conducted along the course of the vessel.

By the first we learn whether the artery has much or little *thickness, hardness and elasticity.*

By the second we are informed as to the degree of *smoothness, of straightness, or of tortuosity; and the elasticity* of the vessel is further tested.

In addition to this form of manipulation, which addresses itself to the arterial walls, there is a *finer fingering* of the pulse itself of which the systematic pressure applied to the artery is but the coarser mode. It can be more easily hinted at than described. It is a touch which tests the qualities of the pulse *through and through*, sometimes playing at the surface, sometimes sounding as it were the depth of the arterial stream, sometimes bearing with full weight against the force of the pulse wave, sometimes pursuing it in its fall and floating up with its rise, a touch as soft and as keen as that of the blind,—in short a touch with a mind in it.

METHODS FOR RAPIDLY FINDING THE PULSATIONS OF SOME OTHER ARTERIES.

How to find the Beat of the Facial Artery.

In this case the distal phalanx (with nail downwards) is brought to bear from above and from the front against the rounded border of the patient's inferior maxilla, immediately anterior to the masseter muscle. *Firm pressure* must be made at first, which will cause the edge of the bone, and perhaps the arterial groove, to be felt. *Pressure is then relaxed* so that the finger remains only in distant touch with the bone, and lies with hardly any weight on the skin. The arterial beat will at once be perceived.

The facility with which this artery is obliterated is very great; indeed it is more apt than the temporal to be unintentionally compressed because although the skin is thicker and better provided with subcutaneous fat, the artery itself, lying in a groove, is in hard bony contact for almost half its circumference.

The artery, as it lies in a loose curve over the slightly convex horizontal surface of the bone, in the angle formed by the masseter and the buccinator muscles, affords an excellent opportunity for some pulse observations.

How to Find the Beat of the Temporal Artery.

It is often necessary to find this beat quickly in an emergency, or during the administration of anæsthetics. Every student should be trained to do this successfully; and with that view the following directions will be found useful.

(1) Whilst you stand behind the patient's head, or at his side, *approach the zygomatic process from below* with the pulp of the median finger turned upwards. The finger is to be gently pressed between the condyle of the jaw below, and the zygoma, the side of the finger just touching the tragus. *Having made firm pressure* so as to feel the border of the bone, *gradually*

reduce the pressure so that the bone is only distantly felt. At this stage the artery will probably be detected. *This is the inferior method.*

FIG. 7.

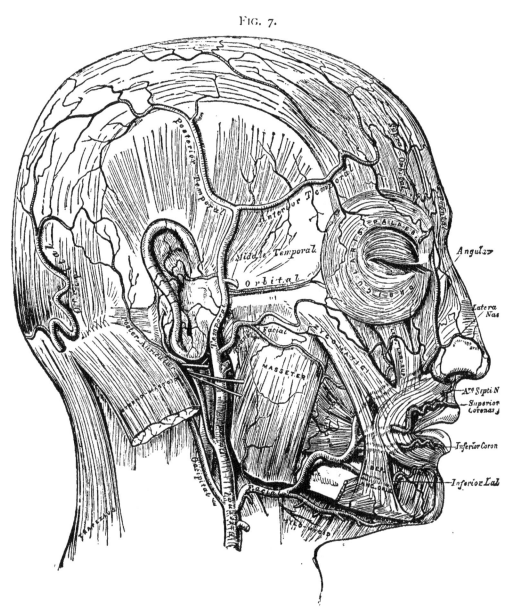

Illustrating the anatomy of the External Carotid, Temporal, Anterior and Posterior Temporal, Facial, Transverse Facial, Coronary, Angular and Occipital Arteries ; and the situations in which their pulsations may be felt.

(*From Gray's " Anatomy," by permission.*)

(2) Exactly analogous is the *superior* method which finds the artery as it crosses the *upper edge of the zygomatic process*.   In this case additional facility is given by the fact that the further course of the artery is superficial, and easilv felt.

FIG. 8.

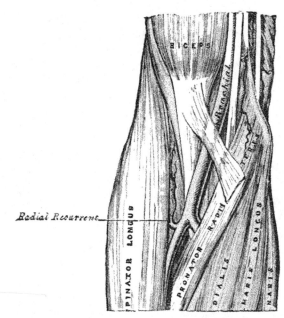

Illustrating the course of the Brachial Artery at the bend of the elbow.

(*From Gray's " Anatomy," by permission.*)

Either of these two methods is to be preferred to the attempt to feel the artery on the dorsum or surface of the zygoma.   Here a very nice adjustment of pressure is necessary.   The artery, being quite superficial and immediately backed by bone without any padding, is readily obliterated in the effort to find it.

How to find the Carotid Beat.

The pulsation of the *common carotid* will be found with great ease, on pressing the tip of the finger *backwards towards the spine, at or above the level of the cricoid cartilage*, and close to its side. The line passing from the horn of the hyoid bone to the tragus roughly corresponds to the course of *the external carotid*, the beat of which is readily felt, although the pressure of the finger is not opposed by any bony surface.

How to find the Brachial Pulse.

Unusually good, and in some ways unique, opportunities for studying the pulse are afforded by the brachial artery. The procedure is so simple that it hardly calls for a special description. The artery is accessible along the entire length of the upper arm. The tip of the finger is *thrust under the biceps from its inner side*, so as gently to lift the muscle with the dorsum of the phalanx, whilst the pulp exerts pressure on the artery *and on the humerus* behind the artery.

CHAPTER II.

ELEMENTARY NOTIONS ON THE PHYSIOLOGY OF THE PULSE.

In this chapter it is proposed very briefly to consider the following subjects for study :—

THE STRUCTURE OF ARTERIES.

THE PULSE-WAVE.

THE INTRA-ARTERIAL BLOOD-PRESSURE.

THE ARTERIAL TENSION.

THE STRUCTURE OF ARTERIES.

All arteries agree in possessing—(1) An *epithelioid* membrane supported by an *elastic membrana propria*. This is the *tunica intima*. (2) A more or less spirally arranged layer of *plain muscular fibres*, supported by a connective-tissue layer. This is the *tunica media*. (3) A *connective-tissue membrane*, consisting mainly of longitudinal bundles and of a varying proportion of elastic fibres. This is the *tunica externa*, which is continuous with the connective tissue surrounding the artery.

In the *larger arteries* (as such we may reckon the radial) the *tunica intima* possesses a much thicker mem brana propria, described, owing to the cribriform arrangement of its elements, as *fenestrated membrane ;* and this membrane, when free from distending pressure, falls into longitudinal wrinkles, seen in transverse sections as festoons.

The media is thick, and consists of alternating muscular and elastic planes united by a small quantity of white connective tissue. The arrangement of the muscular fibres is circular; that of the elastic elements chiefly longitudinal.

The externa contains, besides connective tissue, a quantity of elastic fibres and a few plain muscular fibres. The arrangement is chiefly longitudinal.

The nutrient vessels and the nerves ramify in the externa and penetrate into the media, but not, so far as known, into the intima.

The larger arteries generally possess in addition a tough fibrous sheath containing but little elastic tissue.

The Cardiac Systole and the Pulse-wave.

The systolic charge of the left ventricle, in the adult, is 6 oz. or may vary from 3 to 5 oz. This amount is at each beat of the heart injected with powerful effort into the aorta. The latter, already containing blood, opposes some resistance to the raising of the semilunar valves. The rising intra-ventricular pressure soon disposes of this obstacle and of the resistance offered to further distension by the aortic coats themselves; and a powerful spasm empties the heart.

Two events occur in the arterial system as a result of the systole of the left ventricle:

(1) The *aortic contents are increased, and the aortic stream accelerated;* and

(2) A *wave of pressure is sent through the whole arterial system.*

Inasmuch as the healthy arterial coats are yielding, the wave of increased pressure produces a wave of dilatation of the arterial walls, visible to the naked eye, and appreciable to the touch. *The pulse as it is felt at the wrist is connected with the passage of this wave.*

Velocity of the Pulse-wave.

The velocity of the wave is influenced by various circumstances, but, at its lowest, is still very great (it varies from 16·5 to 33 feet per second).

Velocity of the Blood-stream.

Meanwhile the blood travels in its arterial bed at much slower rates (twenty to thirty times less rapidly).

If, therefore, the radial artery be divided, each spirt (which now takes the place of a pulse) of the arterial jet will belong to the ventricular systole which shall have occurred within the same third of a second; but the *jet itself consists of blood which has left the heart many seconds earlier.*

The velocity of the blood-current varies greatly in the various sections of the vascular system. The following values, taken from Gerald Yeo's "Physiology,"[*] will give some idea of these variations, and from them an estimate may be formed of the average rate of progress of the blood.

Rapidity of Blood-stream.

	Mm. per Second.
Near the Valves of Aorta,—while the ventricles are contracting	1200
In the *Descending Aorta*	300–600
„ *Carotid*	205–357
„ *Radial*	100
„ *Metatarsal*	·57
„ *Arterioles*	50

* Edition 1884, pp. 252, 253.

		Mm. per Second.
In the	*Capillaries*	·5
,,	*Venous Radicles*	25
,,	*Small Veins* on dorsum of hand	50
,,	*Venæ Cavæ*	200

The distinction between pulse-wave and blood-stream having been made clear, the latter need not be again referred to, and subsequent remarks will exclusively apply to the pulse-wave or pressure-wave.

Length of the Pulse-wave.

The length of the pulse-wave is variously estimated by physiologists at 2 *to* 6 *metres*. Prof. Gerald Yeo* says: " Knowing the rate at which the pulse travels (10 m. per sec.) and the time it takes to pass any given point ($\frac{1}{3}$ sec.), its length may be calculated to be about 3 metres, or about twice as long as the longest artery. Thus the pulse-wave reaches the most distant artery in one-sixth of a second, or about the middle of the ventricular systole, and when the wave has passed from the arch of the aorta, its summit has just reached the arterioles." " Hardly more than $\frac{1}{6}$ to $\frac{1}{8}$ of a second lapses between the beat of any two arteries, however distant from each other."

The Pulse-wave, and the Sphygmogram.

A wave travelling at the rate of 20 to 30 feet a second and occupying a length equal to that of two or three men:—this, then. is the pulse-wave. Neither from a casual feel, nor from the sphygmograph, had we gained any idea of these magnitudes, ascertained by experiment. Let us bear them in mind whilst feeling the pulse.

---

* " Manual of Physiology," 2nd edit. 1887, p. 255.

Not only shall we more correctly interpret the sensations conveyed to the finger, but we shall probably feel more than we otherwise should have felt.

The sphygmogram differs so completely from the wave itself that its study is not well fitted to assist our notions of the pulse at the present stage, although invaluable to the advanced student once familiar with the pulse as it is felt.

Intra-arterial Blood-pressure; and Peripheral Resistance.

Arteries during life are always the seat of internal positive pressure. Therefore they not only contain blood at all times, but an amount of blood sufficient to oppose some resistance to the elasticity of the arterial coats.

The existence of a permanent positive pressure is sufficient proof that, whilst the inflow is periodically renewed, the outflow from the arteries is controlled in some permanent manner. This control or impediment is known under the name " peripheral resistance."

The peripheral resistance is made up of—

1. *A more or less constant factor—the friction experienced by the blood-stream in its multitudinous channels;* and

2. *An eminently variable factor—the degree of contraction of the capillaries, and especially of the arterioles.*

From the latter cause variations will arise in the arterial pressure as a result of analogous variations in the peripheral resistance.

The Mean Arterial Pressure.—The Pulse-curves and the Respiratory Undulations of Blood-pressure.

Assuming for a moment that the resistance is steady, the recurring systoles of the heart will cause rhythmic variations of the pressure. *These are termed the " pulse-curves."* Inasmuch as the rise and the fall which they occasion are small, these oscillations do not greatly affect the main level of pressure; and we are able to speak of the *mean arterial pressure* as being steady. The same is true of the rather larger oscillations due to respiration, known as "*respiratory undulations.*" *As soon, however, as the peripheral resistance is altered, whether in plus or in minus, the mean pressure suffers alteration also;* and the circulation as a whole requires re-adjustment. This is brought about in various ways, but chiefly by a modification of the strength of the ventricular systole, and of its frequency.

Amount of the Intra-arterial and Intra-ventricular Pressures.

Measured by the height to which the blood in the artery can lift a column of mercury placed in communication with it, the blood-pressure *in the Brachial Artery (of man) is* 120 *mm.* In the warm-blooded animals the blood-pressure varies (according to the size of each) between 90 mm. and upwards of 200 mm.

The blood-pressure within the *human aorta* has been estimated at 68 oz., or 4 lb. 4 oz. (in the horse it is 11 lb. 9 oz.). In *the human pulmonary artery,* if we were to adopt as correct the generally received statement that the right ventricular wall is one-third thinner than the left, it would be about one-third less. But according to Michael Foster (book i. chap. iv.

p. 253) the pressure within the *right ventricle is probably only* 30 *to* 40 *mm.*, whilst the *left ventricle gives a pressure of* 200 *mm.* Now, this great difference must presumably be proportionate to the difference existing between the peripheral resistance of the pulmonary and that of the systemic circulations, and therefore to the difference between the intra-pulmonary and the intra-aortic pressures. *The radial artery* at the wrist is usually stated to have in health a pressure of 4 dr.

Amount of the Intra-capillary and Intra-venous Blood-pressures.

The capillary blood-pressure can be roughly guessed at, rather than determined, with the help of indirect methods. Thus, in the frog's web a pressure of 11 mm. of mercury is required to exclude the blood from the capillaries. *In the subungual capillaries* of man the pressure requisite varies *from* 20 *to* 30 *mm.*

In the veins, blood-pressure is very low, and becomes lower as the heart is neared. In the larger veins which empty themselves into the thorax it is, during the inspiratory effort, negative or " suctional."

————

ARTERIAL TENSION.

The Artery as an Elastic and Contractile Tube.

Excessive internal pressure will shatter a rigid tube, whilst the same tube, if yielding, would be dilated progressively before rupture. In either case the internal pressure is disposed of in the end owing to the tube giving way. *The arteries likewise are ultimately responsible for the maintenance of the blood-pressure.* They are not rigid. Neither are they merely elastic; for, if so, they might be well adapted for a given degree of pressure, but only imperfectly adapted for any other degree. *Their elasticity is really one capable of a varying pitch, thanks to the regulating influence of the muscular coat.* Moreover, the elasticity of an artery is, in some proportion, made up of the elasticity proper to its muscular fibres; and this is essentially subject to variations. In a word, arteries are contractile as well as elastic.

Varying Calibre and Arterial Tension.—"Softness" and "Hardness" of Pulse.

So long as the muscular fibres do not contract we may regard the artery as an ordinary elastic tube possessing a definite resistance and power of recoil. Whenever the fibres contract, whether much or little, the lumen or calibre will of course be altered; at the same time, however, the thickness of the arterial wall will vary, and also its resistance and its elasticity.

Let us consider *any one* of the numerous sizes of which an artery is capable. Just as an india-rubber air-cushion may be inflated much or little, and will become, according to the degree of inflation, tense and hard, or soft and lax, so will the arterial wall be more or less stretched by the blood within. As the tension rises, its surface will become more and more rigid and hard, so that little remains of its natural quality of softness; neither will the mobile properties by which we are able to recognise the presence of fluid be any longer perceived.

Independently, therefore, of the size, *the softness or*

hardness of the arterial surface may become a guide to the degree of the blood-pressure.

Influence of Elasticity on Arterial Tension.

The elasticity of the artery we may compare to a *buffer*, inasmuch as it fulfils a double object—(1) that of protecting the part subjected to pressure, viz., the arterial wall : (2) that of storing up energy to be employed in · propelling the blood as soon as the pressure is no longer in excess. In other words, it saves the artery from the danger of rupture and it assists the heart in keeping up the general circulation.

From that which has preceded it may be gathered that, the greater the systolic pressure, so much the more energy will be stored up. For a moment this energy is held in check by the same resistance which was the means of causing the pressure to rise ; and the artery will collapse only *by degrees* in proportion as the resist ance becomes reduced.

It is thus explained why, under ordinary circumstances, *arterial tension, if it be great, will also be sus tained.* Conversely, if small, it will correspond to a small blood-pressure and peripheral resistance ; and also to a small store of elastic energy, which will be *quickly* expended in overcoming the small obstacle. Thus *low arterial tensions will not be long sustained.*

Dicrotism.

In some thin persons, if the wrist be held up to a powerful light, each pulse-wave may be seen to experience during its fall a momentary check, as though it would swing up again to its previous position. *It is this secondary wave or beat which has given rise to the name Dicrotism. The normal pulse may be dicrotic;* but this feature is not often so sharply marked as to be felt by the finger. A keen eye will, however, detect it in *relaxed arteries*, the seat of *low tension.*

In Fever, when the arterial walls are relaxed by heat and the blood-tension is low, whilst the heart is working with short and frequent systoles, a careful touch on the radial artery will easily realise the dicrotic jerk, which is then much more prominent than in the normal state.

Dicrotism was observed under these circumstances before the days of the sphygmograph. But we owe to the latter the discovery that the dicrotic event occurs also in the healthy pulse-wave. The student will have no difficulty in detecting dicrotism in fever; but only very close attention will enable him to trace it, when present, in the normal pulse; this is an exercise the practice of which cannot fail to educate his touch in a very high degree.

The Arterial Foot-jerk as a Type of the Sphygmograph.

The dicrotic wavelet is much more readily detected in the larger arteries than in the radial. It is well for this reason to investigate the axillary, the brachial, the femoral, and the popliteal pulses. The last named affords a very good ocular demonstration of the pulse-wave and of its dicrotism when *one leg is crossed over the opposite knee.* If the supported limb be allowed to hang loosely, the foot may be observed to oscillate with each cardiac systole. The jerk of the popliteal pulse-wave is in this case multiplied by the length of the swinging limb ; and a writing lever suitably fixed to the foot could be made to yield a tracing of the pulse.

This simple experiment gives a complete demonstration of the principle and of the essential factors of the sphygmograph :

(1) *The weight of the limb represents the* **pressure** *applied to the artery ;*

(2) *The leg plays the part of the* **lever ;** *and*

(3) *The action of the* **spring** *is supplied by the gravitation of the foot back to its position of rest after each pulse-jerk.*   The dicrotic or secondary jerk is in this case rendered very conspicuous.

CHAPTER III.

THE CHIEF QUALITIES AND VARIETIES OF THE NORMAL PULSE.

——•◦•——

Individual Variety Considerable.—Importance of a Systematic Study of Large Numbers of Pulses.

THERE. are certain limits beyond which the exaggeration of some one feature of the pulse becomes an abnormality. But within these boundaries there is space for a very large variety of combinations; so much so that it would be difficult to meet with two persons in whom the radial pulse was exactly alike. This endless variety is a source of difficulty in describing to our satisfaction the pulse such as it is felt in any individual case. It accounts for the large assortment of adjectives and for the startling array of figures of speech which have been called to our aid (some of these will be found in the Glossary), and makes it evident that experience is the only means to a comprehensive knowledge of the pulse.

Let the student note, however, that a *large experience is not necessarily a long one.* Nay, it may be held that multiple observations compressed within a short space of time would probably lead to a better and more definite perception of the varieties in type than the same number of impressions spread over intervals too long to render comparison easy. He has an opportunity that he would do well to utilize at an early period of his clinical studies, to systematically feel *a considerable number of normal pulses, and to compare at first such large categories as the senile, the adult, and the puerile pulses; the male and the female pulse; the pulse of short and of high stature, &c.* By degrees he will rise to a capacity for discerning finer distinctions; and when his attention is turned to the study of disease he will find himself competent to observe and to describe wherein any pulse may be abnormal.

SYSTEMATIC DESCRIPTION OF THE QUALITIES OF THE PULSE

In these pages a similar process is adopted. We will proceed to analyse the pulse, that is, to consider one by one the physical qualities which make themselves known to us, and which alone we are capable of describing accurately. Every pulse will have to be studied on this basis at first,—just as an artist's first sketch is built up on anatomical lines. Coarse differences between pulses will be brought to light by the method, but the finer touches which will make the description so like the original as to convey a complete mental picture of it can hardly be expected at an early stage of study.

Large and Small Size or Volume of Pulse.

A "large pulse" and a "small pulse" are expressions which appeal to any person who has compared with each other a few examples of the healthy pulse. All beginners are exposed to the risk of getting an inadequate idea of the size of the radial pulse from not having sufficiently relaxed the tendons with which it is surrounded. If this be done, that which appeared previously to be a small pulse may be ultimately recognised as a relatively large one.

The largest "volume" of pulse results from a combination of two factors:

1. *A strong heart-beat*, and
2. *A yielding arterial wall, alike capable of collapse and of distension.*

Conversely, a small pulse would be found in those whose arteries were not so yielding, or the heart so strong.

It must be noted, however, that an artery may be large and yet very unyielding when the superior power of the heart has gradually brought about general arterial dilatation.

As a broad statement; it is true to say that a *"large pulse" is generally infrequent; a small pulse, frequent.*

So-called "Fulness" and "Emptiness" of Pulse.

"Fulness" and "emptiness," when applied to the pulse, are expressions almost entirely metaphorical. *Arteries are never empty during life,* although they may contain much less blood at one time than at another. In truth, arteries *adapt their size* to their contents, and in that sense they are always full. Any tendency to a vacuum, if it existed, would produce a collapse of their walls; and at the same time would act as a negative or suctional force, detaining the blood within them.

By "full pulse" is presumably meant *a stout and firm pulse*, not readily subsiding; by "empty pulse," *one quickly vanishing* after a spasmodic beat. Here again we should gain in clearness by avoiding the words " full " and " empty " and using the equivalents which more truly correspond to the things as they are.

" Strength " and " Weakness " of Pulse-wave.

It is much less clear what meaning should be attached to the terms " strong " and " weak " pulse. Nothing is more probable in appearance than that a considerable rise and expansion of the artery should mean a powerful cardiac systole, and therefore a strong pulse. Often enough this is the case. *Very frequently, however, the size of the pulse is not a reliable measure of its strength.* The large and full pulsation is apt to be very short and one easily compressed. Resistance, on the other hand, is often a character of pulses whose beats are not tall, and which possess but moderate volume. We shall therefore connect the expression strong and weak rather with the *lifting power* of the pulse-wave than with the degree of expansion or height of rise special to the individual beats when no external pressure is superadded.

The paradox apparently implied in the association of contradictory terms, such as " *large* pulse of *small* strength," will be partly explained away by later remarks on arterial tension, but it may even at this stage be pointed out that the smaller size which a pulsation may possess sometimes coincides with very powerful cardiac effort, and with considerable strength, just as a spiral spring partly weighted down by a heavy load, nevertheless gives us proof of greater power than we can be sure of in the taller spring which no weight has yet tried.

Let us be very careful, therefore, in every case of

large pulsation to try the effect of a strong pressure of the finger, and to notice the relative duration of the pulse-wave, and the condition of the artery in the intervals between successive waves.

The Artery during the Interval between Beats.

Hitherto we have referred only to the strength of the pulsation. Shifting now the ground of our observation from the pulsation to the condition of the *artery between successive beats* we shall find that, among the large pulses, some persist during the interval whilst others fade away after the systolic jerk.* *The first set are strong as well as large pulses; the second, weak in spite of their large size.* Conversely, a small pulse may become imperceptible between the beats; it is then weak as well as small. But it may be strong although small, if during the intervals it resist the ordinary attempts at compression.

Softness and Hardness of Pulse.

"Softness" and "hardness" are qualities of which the touch is an accurate judge: the words in this case are truly descriptive. *A pulse may be hard from undue pressure of its fluid contents, or from undue solidification of the arterial walls.* It is not always easy to tell whether the hardness is due to blood-pressure or to tissue condensation of the arterial surface. Both these variations occur as a *senile change*. A *soft pulse* is produced when the arterial walls are free

---

* These remarks apply to pulses in general, not to the pathological variety known as Corrigan's pulse, in which the beat is forcible, but ends abruptly.

from thickening, and the blood is free from undue pressure. Softness and elasticity (during the periods of bodily and mental rest) are attributes of a *juvenile pulse*.

Elasticity of Pulse.

Arteries in health are both yielding and very elastic. Age sooner or later impairs the natural elasticity and expansibility of the vessels. The same regressive change may also result from disease, independently of age.

The presence of the elastic property is easily recognised in *the recoil* of the artery after each pulsation. Its absence, where this recoil does not take place. is more difficult to prove; the systolic pressure in some individuals, and at some times, is so great and so long sustained that the elastic force of the artery is overpowered. Elasticity is then not necessarily extinct; it may be simply latent because maintained on the stretch. The strain which this implies is considerable, and it could not be kept up for protracted periods without lasting impairment and ultimate destruction of the elastic property.

Swiftness and Slowness of Pulse; or Short and Long Duration of the Pulse-wave.

A swift pulse is one rapidly passing from the period of arterial expansion to that of collapse. This certainly means that *the wave travels fast ;* it may, in addition, mean that *its length is reduced.* Rapidity of the pulse-wave is usually associated with frequency of rate. The reverse is the case with the *slow pulsation, which is commonly an infrequent one.* Swiftness is almost invariably, no less than frequency, *the · result of diminished peripheral resistance;* and, conversely, slowness and infrequency indicate an abnormal obstacle, occurring somewhere in the arterial or in the capillary circulation. *Contraction of the arterioles* constitutes an obstacle of this kind. A well-known instance is the contraction of the cutaneous vessels as a result of cold. *Rigidity of the arteries,* as in senile thickening of their coats, is another form of increased resistance, more serious than the first, because permanent and progressive.

Frequency and Infrequency of Pulse; or Pulse-rate.

No uncertainty can possibly attach to the use of these expressions. They correspond to the old Latin terms *pulsus creber, pulsus rarus.* They are much to be preferred to the words " rapid " and " slow," which are applicable to the rate of progress of the pulse-wave as well as to the rate at which the cardiac beats succeed each other. Nevertheless, the expressions " quick," " fast," or " rapid pulse "—and " slow pulse " have passed into currency, and are generally understood to apply to the pulse-rate. It is worth while, however, to be absolutely correct in this matter for the sake of complete clearness, and *to speak, not of the " pulse," but of the " pulse-rate," as being either slow or fast.*

Accelerating and Retarding Influences.

The causes which accelerate the pulse-rate are many, and a majority of them are *physiological.* Among the latter may be specially mentioned *physical exertion, psychical excitement, and external heat.*

Pathologically, an increase in the pulse-rate is bound

up with a rise in the internal, or body-temperature, in fever. Apart from fever, it is often witnessed as a result of disordered nerve-function, and as a mechanical consequence of various forms of heart disease.

On the contrary, **infrequency of pulse** is more often due to pathological than to physiological causes. It is true that during rest, and especially in healthy sleep, the heart slackens speed. Again, with some individuals, a remarkable slowness of the heart-rate is "natural" or "constitutional." Of this the most famous historical instance is that of the great Napoleon, whose pulse-rate is stated to have been habitually 40. More commonly, however, infrequency is the result of some definite abnormality, whether cardiac or vascular. A very slow pulse-rate is often witnessed in *fatty degeneration of the heart*, but slowness is by no means invariably present in this disease. Sometimes an abnormally slow pulse-rate is the result of excessive *feebleness of some of the heart-beats*, whereby they are unable to reach the periphery (see Abortive Beats and Linked Beats).

Putting aside the exceptional cases just mentioned, a determination of the pulse-rate is so easy of performance that this subject has been very thoroughly investigated. The following are the results, some of which are familiar to every student of physiology :—

I. The Normal Rate in the Two Sexes.

The normal frequency per minute is—

> 72 in the adult male,
> 80 in the adult female ;

(according to Ozanam, respectively 60 and 70).

II. Influence of Age.

The pulse-rate varies with age in the following manner :—

Pulse-rate in the fœtus	.	.	.	.	.		140–150
,,	,,	at birth	.	.	.	.	.	130–140
,,	,,	at 1 year of age		.	.	.	.	120–130
,,	,,	at 2 years of age		.	.	.	.	105
,,	,,	at 3 ,, ,,	:	:	:	:	:	100
,,	,,	at 4 ,, ,,		.	.	.	.	97
,,	,,	at 5 ,, ,,		.	.	.	.	94–90
,,	,,	at 10 ,, ,,			about			90
,,	,,	from 10 to 15 years of age						78
,,	,,	from 15 to 50 ,, ,,						70
,,	,,	at 60 years of age	.	.	.	.		74
,,	,,	at 80 ,, ,,		.	.	.	.	79
,,	,,	from 80 to 90 .	.		upwards of			80

According to the above figures, which are taken from Stirling's translation of Landois' Physiology, it will be seen that, in the adult, *any pulse-rate between the rates of* 60 *and* 80 *pulsations per minute might be regarded as a normal rate, any rate below* 60 *might be regarded as a slow rate, any rate above* 90 *might be regarded as a quick rate.*

III. The Influence of Stature.

The influence of *body-length* is to lessen the frequency of pulse and to increase the blood-pressure.

Czarnecki derived the following results with the help of the formulæ of Volkmann and Rameaux · *

Height.	Rate.	Calculated.	Height.	Rate.	Calculated.
80–90 cm. .	103	90	140–150 cm.	74	69
90–100	91	86	150–160	68	67
100–110	87	81	160–170 .	65	65
110–120	84	78	170–180 ·	64	63
120–130	78	75	above 180	60	60
130–140 .	76 ...	72			

* See Landois' Physiology, translated by Stirling, 1885, p. 142.

IV. The Influence of the Hour of Day.

The following figures are given by Landois in connection with variations in frequency ·

3–6 A.M.	61 pulsations.
8–11½ A.M.	74 „
11½–2 P.M.	a fall.
3 P.M. (dinner-time) and till 6 or 8 P.M. a rise to 70	„
8–12 P.M.	a fall to 54 „

Thus the maximum is in the forenoon, the minimum at midnight.

V. The Influence of Sleep and the Waking State.

The preceding table shows that sleep is accompanied by a slow rate of heart-beat and that the quickest rate belongs to the hours of complete wakefulness and activity. Moreover, the act of awaking is associated with a rise in the pulse-rate, the more marked if the awakening be abrupt and not spontaneous.

VI. The Influence of Meals and of the Fasting State.

The pulse is kept low as well as slow, by fasting. It is accelerated, and at the same time excited, by meals (*febris a prandio*).

VII. The Influence of the Quantity and of the Quality of Food.

The acceleration brought about by a large meal is greater than that due to a small one, and it is maintained for two or three hours. But the variety and especially the temperature of the food have very distinct effects on the pulse, irrespective of quantity. Warm foods, and especially warm drinks, immediately raise the pulse-rate; cold food or drinks only after a while (Ozanam). Vinegar, sour milk, fruit are said to depress the pulse-rate. The acceleration due to nitrogenous foods is less delayed, but that due to non-nitrogenous foods lasts longer.

Alcohol, Tea, and Coffee.

The accelerating action of these beverages is too familiar to call for comment. In the case of tea or coffee it is said to disappear within an hour, but, as is well known, individual susceptibility varies greatly.

VIII. The Influence of Tobacco-smoking.

According to Nick (quoted by Ozanam), acceleration is produced even in those who have acquired the habit. The increase of pulse-rate occasioned by smoking a pipe of tobacco in the morning "may amount to from 15 to 20 pulsations, and last an hour."

IX. The Influence of Muscular Exercise and of Rest.

Rest slows the pulse; muscular exercise invariably quickens it; roughly speaking, in proportion to the amount of the exertion. This subject was carefully studied by Nick (1831). His interesting results are in harmony with modern physiological data.

X. The Influence of Posture.

What has just been said almost implies that attitudes will influence the rapidity of the pulse in proportion to the muscular effort which they necessitate. This was proved to be the case by Guy. Standing up, being much more laborious than sitting up, accelerates the pulse in a

greater measure than the latter; and it may be due to
the fact that there is more energy in the usual attitude
of a man than in that of a woman that this acceleration
is less in the latter than in the former.

XI. The Influence of Emotion, of Psychical and of Mental Excitement.

The usual effect is an acceleration; but in some cases
emotion, especially if it be of the nature of a severe
shock to the feelings, produces slowing and at the same
time temporary feebleness of the heart's beat (faintness
and fainting).

The influence of the psychical and sensorial factors
is shown in the *increase in pulse-rate* and blood-pressure
induced in animals as well as in man *by music.*

XII. The Influence of Variations in Barometric Pressure.

Although slight oscillations in the atmospheric
pressure do not perceptibly alter the pulse-rate, this
influence is very marked when the changes in pressure
are considerable.   Thus, at high altitudes, the pulse
beats at a much increased rate; and, conversely, at low
levels, such as that of the Dead Sea (430 metres below
the sea-level) or in deep mines, the rhythm of the heart
is much slowed (Ozanam).

XIII. The Influence of Variations in the External Temperature.

*Heat accelerates the heart's action; cold diminishes the
rate.*   It is owing to this agency that inhabitants of a
cold climate have a slower pulse than the inhabitants
of tropical regions (Ozanam).   A practical demonstra-

tion of this effect of external heat is readily obtained in the hot-room of a Turkish bath.

XIV The Influence of Variations in the Temperature of the Body.

Whenever the body heat sinks below the normal, the rapidity of the heart's action (*cæteris paribus*) is diminished. On the contrary, a rise above the normal temperature is accompanied by acceleration. The quick pulse-rate in fever is in great part due to this cause, and the acceleration is proportionate to the rise. According to Sir William Aitken, a rise of one degree Fahrenheit corresponds very closely to an increase of 10 pulsations per minute.

CHAPTER IV.

THE CHIEF ABNORMALITIES OF THE PULSE.

In this chapter are briefly considered :

  I. *The variations in size.*
  II. *The variations in rhythm.*
  III. *The incompressible pulse ;* and
  IV. *The recurrent pulse.*

On the Use of the Terms "Irregularity" and "Unevenness."

Regularity in the intervals, and equality in the beats, are essential features of the normal pulse. In disturbed function either one or the other or even both may be affected. Since alterations of this kind are of common occurrence, clearness would best be served by the use of two distinct terms. Although irregularity may be understood to apply both to disturbances in time and to variations in strength ; yet *unevenness* is specially suggestive of alterations in level, and most fitly expresses the broken line formed by the summits of unequal pulse-waves. Without unfair restriction and with great advantage we may therefore reserve the terms "*uneven pulse*" *for the condition of unequal pulse beats,* and "*irregular pulse*" *for disturbance of rhythm, or arhythmia.* The strength of pulsations, as well as their frequency, are subject to fluctuations according to the time of day and to its events; it is necessary, therefore, to state that " irregularity " and " unevenness " would be applicable only to changes more rapid than these.

I.

THE VARIATIONS IN SIZE.

" Unevenness " of Pulse.

In health the *size of the pulse* is subject only to the physiological variations previously described. It maintains a uniform level so long as no changes occur in the external circumstances. In some persons, however healthy according to appearances and as regards their own feelings, the *heart acts unevenly;* in them the unevenness is almost always associated with irregularity of pulse. Although the general strength need not suffer, we recognise in this symptom evidence of disordered function. Cases of this kind strikingly illustrate the meaning of *functional as contrasted with organic disease.* In the latter, unevenness arises as a result of anatomical changes in the heart or its valves, and has a widely different significance. The unevenness and irregularity special to the purely nervous affections are often alarming to the patient when first discovered by him; and even to the observer accustomed to meet with them, there is always something strange in the sensation which they convey; for rhythm and evenness are natural to organic life and their absence is disquieting even when it is not dangerous.

Unevenness in pulse has two distinct types·

(1) *The unevenness may be periodic, and in this sense regular; or*

(2) *it may follow no definite rule.*

Periodic Unevenness.

Of this we sometimes meet with striking examples. *Pulsus alternans* is characterised by unevenness in the size of every other beat. It is a good instance of the unusual *combination of regularity in rhythm, with unevenness in size.* The relative value of the two beats in *pulsus alternans* varies in different cases. The smaller beat, should it be very small, may be "abortive," *i.e.,* may not reach the wrist with sufficient force to be felt. The radial pulse will be regular but its rate will then be half the rate of the cardiac pulsation.

In *pulsus bigeminus* the beats run in pairs, between which a relatively long interval occurs.

Pulsus trigeminus, even less common than the preceding form, resembles it in the long intervals which separate groups of pulsations. Each group in this case consists of three beats.

Abortive Beats.

An instance of single abortive beats has been given in connection with *pulsus alternans.* Two or even three abortive beats may succeed one strong beat. This occurs in a good percentage of the cases of very slow pulse. Commonly the *accessory beats* are so small that even the stethoscope may fail to render them plainly audible, and they may be but feebly indicated in the sphygmographic pulse-tracing.

Non-Periodic Unevenness.

Often abortive beats are isolated and occur at irregular intervals. In this case the finger resting on the *pulse* would notice a sudden blank followed by a return to the normal rhythm. But if the *heart's action* had meanwhile been under observation with the binaural stethoscope, two events would have been noticed: (1) an *unusually early, unusually short* and *spasmodic beat*, seeming to overtake the preceding beat (just as in tripping or stumbling, one foot is hurriedly brought forward to save a fall); (2) an unusually long pause. This, taken together with the short beat, is nearly equivalent to the added durations of one ordinary beat and two ordinary pauses.

Linked Beats.

Instead of one there may be two abortive beats rapidly succeeding one another, and followed by a long pause. Both in this case and in the preceding one the group formed by the large beat and the small beats receives the name of linked pulsations.

Difference between Linked Beats and Pulsus Bigeminus and Trigeminus.

It often occurs that the linked beats are felt at the wrist, as well as heard at the heart. The student will have no difficulty in knowing them and putting upon them the correct name if he will bear in mind that, in the other variety (the *pulsus bigeminus* and *trigeminus* of Traube), the size of the beats in each group is nearly, if not quite equal; *they are complete beats.* In *linked beats* this is not the case; the second beat occurs before the natural end of the previous one; and whilst curtailing this, it is itself much hurried and very imperfect.

The term *stumbling or tripping pulsation* describes the irregular and spasmodic heart's action which causes the linked beats. It is applicable to the pulse as well as to the heart's action.

Combined Unevenness and Irregularity.

Absolute unevenness, associated with absolute irregularity, is a common form of functional disturbance. Among the valvular affections it is distinctive, although not exclusively so, of *mitral regurgitation*, particularly in its worst form and in its later stages. Instances of this combination have been alluded to under the head of abortive and linked beats.

II.

THE VARIATIONS IN RHYTHM.

"Irregularity" of Pulse.   Intermittence.
Allorhythmia and Arhythmia.

The remarks made in connection with unevenness of the pulse give prominence to the fact that an uneven pulse is most commonly irregular also. Even in those instances where periodicity is traceable in the recurrence of unequal beats, the rhythm is altered (*allorhythmia*) though it is not quite destroyed. Indeed, if the heart's action alone were under consideration, it might be truly said that marked unevenness is always coupled with irregularity, and *vice versâ*.

In the radial pulse, however, the cardiac events are not always faithfully represented. Slightly uneven systoles are in a measure equalised by the elasticity of the intervening arteries. On the other hand, very feeble systoles are often not conveyed as pulse-beats as far as the wrist. It will often happen, therefore, that the radial pulse will be very irregular in rhythm without any proportionate unevenness in its beats. Thus we may, without doing any violence to facts, award a separate consideration to the subject of irregularity.

Intermittence and Allorhythmia.

There are two types of irregularity :

1. *The pulse rhythm may be suddenly interrupted* by a pause of greater duration than normal. The pulse is then said to be *intermittent*. This is the common form.

2. The pulse, whilst not suffering any stoppage, may *suddenly undergo acceleration or slowing*, It is then said to be *allorhythmic*.

Both these forms of irregularity may be periodic or non-periodic, and we shall have four varieties to consider.

1. *The periodic or regular intermittence.*

2. *The irregular intermittence.*

3. *The periodic or regular allorhythmia.*

4. *The non-periodic or irregular allorhythmia.*

We may at once dismiss the last two varieties as not possessing at the present stage any practical interest, and confine our attention to the intermittent pulse.

Intermittence at the Wrist.

As previously hinted, the dropping of a beat at the wrist may mean very different cardiac events. This is clearly shown by what has been said under the heading " Abortive Beats."

One of three things may have happened :

1. *The missing beat may never have been given by the heart. (Intermittence at the heart.)*

2. *It may have been a feeble heart-beat*, of the nature of the weaker beat in *pulsus alternans*, and too feeble to be felt at the wrist

3. *It may have been of the nature of a linked beat* (hurried and incomplete, and too early as well as too short).

The first of these conditions, namely—*cardiac inter mittence*—is the most common, as a cause for intermittence at the wrist.

The Varieties of Rhythm in Intermittence.

Although it is important to hold fast by the distinction between the regular and the irregular intermissions, we are not at present in possession of definite knowledge as to the relative value of the two classes of events as regards either diagnosis or prognosis. The degree of the abnormality would seem to be more important than the kind; and yet in some cases the irregularity may be considerable without any apparent detriment to health or capacity for work. (The most common association and the most probable cause of this peculiarity is dyspepsia in some form or other; such, at least, is the current opinion.) Nevertheless, in the clinical study of cases it is most desirable to discover and note any periodicity which may exist, or to ascertain that, on the contrary, the intermittence is subject to no definite rhythm.

Absolute Arhythmia.

Outside the large group of functional (usually dyspeptic) cases to which reference has been made, *complete arhythmia* (absolute irregularity) is met with in cases of cardiac exhaustion, and during the agony of death by gradual heart failure. This fact contains the suggestion, which was successfully put to the test by Knoll,[*] that irregularities such as *pulsus bigeminus* and *trigeminus*, and arhythmia in general, might be induced by casting upon the heart an amount of work disproportionate to its energy. Complete arhythmia is always coupled with a high degree of unevenness of beat.

Classical Varieties of Uneven and Irregular Pulse, known under Special Names.

Under this heading we shall proceed to a short account of the following varieties :—

1. *Pulsus inciduus,*
2. *Pulsus myurus,*
3. *Pulsus paradoxus.*

The old names, *pulsus inciduus, pulsus myurus,* both apply to unevenness of pulse. *Pulsus paradoxus* is both uneven and irregular.

Pulsus inciduus, or *waxing and waning pulse,* consists of successive short periods of pulsations, beginning with a strong beat, and, after gradual diminution, ending with a weak beat.

In **pulsus myurus**—a pathological curiosity—the pulse strength gradually tapers away " like the tail of a rat." In former days the practice of bleeding *ad animæ dereliquium usque* afforded frequent opportunities for feeling this form of pulse. It may also be observed in the umbilical artery at birth whilst the placental circulation is being diverted.

Pulsus Paradoxus, cum Inspiratione Intermittens.

The pulsus paradoxus may be regarded as a special variety of *pulsus inciduus,* in which—

---

[*] See Landois' Physiology, translated by Stirling, edition 1885, p. 143.

(*a*) The unevenness coincides with, and is dependent upon, the movements of respiration, and

(*b*) The beats may be so much reduced as to cease to be felt at the wrists

The cardiac rhythm and blood-pressure are *normally* influenced by respiration, *the rate decreasing slightly and the pressure increasing during inspiration*, whilst the reverse takes place during expiration.* The variety described as paradoxical by Kussmaul, presents, on the contrary, *an inspiratory fall* of pressure in the peripheral arteries.

Normally, the inspiratory negative pressure within the thorax takes effect upon the subclavian arteries, and, according to Marey, upon the aorta itself. This would tend to lower, during inspiration, the pressure within the arteries of the upper limb. But, in opposition to this result, a *stronger influence prevails under ordinary circumstances—namely, that of the increased in-take of venous blood by the heart during early inspiration*. It is clear, however, that any cause which would intensify thoracic aspiration beyond a certain point, must lead to an inspiratory fall of pressure. The strong efforts of dyspnœa in cases where the lungs, owing to the presence of fluid effusions, tumours, adhesions, infiltration, or stenosis of the air-passages, were unable to expand, would take excessive action of this kind on the heart and large vessels, and influence the pulse in the paradoxical direction. But in these cases the heart-sounds would be altered as regards time and strength.

Implication of the heart does not occur in the *special form described by Kussmaul*. In this variety, whilst

---

* See Landois' Physiology, translated by Stirling, edition 1885, p. 148.

the pulse falters, the *heart rate and strength of beat are not modified*. It is therefore manifest that the influence at work is not one having its seat *at* the heart, but *beyond it*. The first case of *pulsus paradoxus* described by Kussmaul* occurred in a patient affected with *callous mediastino-pericarditis* (*of Griesinger*) and the symptoms in this patient were explained by the existence of a *fibrous constriction* of the large vessels. The fibrous bands, becoming tense during inspiration, occasioned increasing compression and temporary stoppage of the pulse with each breath. Intermittent pressure on the great vessels may be set up in a similar way by a variety of causes.

Before taking leave of this subject, it should be mentioned that an analogous influence has been traced by Marev† in cases of intra-thoracic aneurysm, the blood-pressure falling during each inspiratory phase.

III.

THE INCOMPRESSIBLE PULSE—SO-CALLED.

Very rarely indeed can a pulse be correctly termed incompressible. In dealing with this question we must regard any unusual resistance offered by the pulse as due to the condition of the artery itself, considered as a tube, or to the pressure of its contents.

(1) *As regards blood-pressure.* Much force may have to be opposed by the finger to the *vis a tergo* propagated from the ventricle, and to the resulting distension of the artery between the beats, before the resistance is over-

---

* *Berl. Klin. Wochenschr.*, 1873, No. 37–39.
† "Circulation du Sang," 1887, p. 643.

come. But in the grasp of a healthy man there is much more power than is necessary for this end. *Therefore blood-pressure, however high, is never in itself sufficient to render a pulse incompressible.*

(2) *As regards the arterial wall*, it must be borne in mind that thin tubes, such as an india-rubber tube, originally soft, may through age become so stiffened and hardened as to break rather than bend under pressure; any tube of this kind would, in a sense, be incompressible. Again, tubes made of a very dense material, such as glass, clay, or metal, will, in spite of their thinness, defy the strongest pressure that the finger can put upon them; these tubes likewise are incompressible.

Arterial Sclerosis.

Now, arteries in general are liable to changes tending to make them resemble either one or the other of the above-mentioned varieties of incompressible tubing, or even both varieties at once. Thus, they may become *sclerosed,* in other words, *thickened and stiffened;* but owing to their perpetual exercise by the heart's recurring systole, they never become set. They may feel firm, thick, and leathery; and may in a measure *resist* compression; but they are never from this cause alone incompressible.

Calcification of the Arterial Wall.

In addition, arteries may become *partly solidified owing to the deposition of calcareous particles*, in which case, the deposition being progressive, absolute rigidity is a conceivable result. It is unusual, however, for the calcification to proceed evenly along any considerable length of the vessel; and between the calcareous islands the artery preserves some of its original pliability. The conversion of a radial artery into anything comparable to the stem of a clay pipe is therefore very rare ; and its absolute incompressibility should be classed among the most unlikely contingencies. But the rings or patches of calcification may be so extensive and so close set as to render the artery *relatively incompressible,* the amount of force by which its rigidity might be overcome being undesirable or even dangerous to apply.

In conclusion, a high degree of calcification is the only cause which would render incompressible an artery whose channel was still pervious and large ; and, the range of operation of this cause being limited to those advanced in years, *incompressibility,* truly so called, is of rare occurrence.

Most pulses alleged to be incompressible are not so in reality. The cause of the erroneous impression we shall now proceed to explain, in connection with recurrent pulsation.

IV

The Recurrent Pulse.

Circulation by Anastomosis.

In peripheral districts of the circulation, whenever the channel of an artery is accidentally blocked by a locally developed (thrombotic) or by an imported (embolic) clot, or by a surgical ligature, the blood, checked in its direct passage, finds a circuitous way, by anastomosis, into the distal segment. If the channel of communication be through fairly large arteries, pulsation will appear, *after a short interval* or *immediately*, in the distal segment; and in this the pulse-wave will *travel backwards, towards the heart.* This is the usual sequence after ligature for aneurysm.

Refluent Radial Pulse.

Precisely the same events may occur when the radial artery is compressed in feeling the pulse. If digital pressure were kept up for a sufficient time, recurrent pulsation would ultimately be developed in all subjects tried as to this peculiar phenomenon, but probably after varying delays.

Fig. 9.

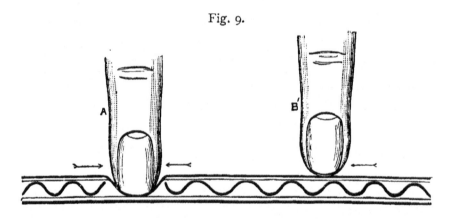

Illustrating recurrent pulsation at B′, after complete obliteration of the pulse at A. (Reproduced with Dr. Douglas Powell's kind permission.)

In some persons no delay occurs. No sooner is the finger firmly pressed down on the artery so as to stop the pulse-wave, than another wave rushes up under the testing finger placed a little further down on the course of the artery. These facts are excellently illustrated in the accompanying diagrams, reproduced from Dr. Douglas Powell's paper on "Angina Pectoris, its Nature and Treatment" (in the Medical Society's *Transactions,* vol. xiv.), with the author's kind permission.   In cases of this kind, try what we will, pulsation persists

" tamen usque recurrit."

In a word, the pulse is *unsuppressed*.

Nevertheless, proof may be obtained that the artery has been *effectually compressed and obliterated* by finger A; and that the pulsation detected by finger B' reaches it from the periphery.   This is best done by the method suggested by Dr. Douglas Powell, and illustrated in his second diagram (see Fig. 10).   If a

Fig. 10.

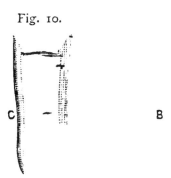

Illustrating the mode in which the pulse may be tested as to its complete obliteration by pressure.   (Reproduced with Dr. Douglas Powell's kind permission.)

third finger (c) be placed between the other two, whilst powerful pressure is made on the artery by both of these alike, no pulsation will be felt by the finger c. A glance at Fig. 1, p. 11, will remind the reader of the collateral channel through which the recurrent pulse-wave takes its course.

CHAPTER V.

THE SIX CHIEF MORBID PULSE TYPES.
HOW TO TEST THE PULSE AS TO TENSION.

THE chief morbid varieties of pulse usually require no sphygmograph for their diagnosis. The student should not rest till he has been given an opportunity of feeling each of the following typical pulses of disease :—

(1) *The pulse of abnormally high arterial tension,*
(2) *The pulse of abnormally low arterial tension,*
(3) *The pulse of mitral regurgitation,*
(4) *The pulse of mitral obstruction,*
(5) *The pulse of aortic regurgitation,*
(6) *The pulse of aortic obstruction.*

To these might have been added *the pulse of hypertrophy* and *the pulse of dilatation.* These, however, unless unusually pronounced, are not, on the one hand, sharply marked off from some of the extreme variations of the pulse in health ; neither do they greatly differ, on the other hand, from some of the other morbid pulses.

PRELIMINARY DESCRIPTION OF THE METHODS FOR GAUGING ARTERIAL TENSION WITH THE FINGER.

Whenever it is necessary *to determine with precision* the strength of the pulse-wave and the tension of the radial artery, recourse must be had to the *sphygmo-graph*, a description of which we have not attempted in these elementary pages. With the help of that instrument both the strength and the tension can be made out in a satisfactory manner. In medical practice, however, information as to the tension of pulse in cases of illness is a need of every hour, although more than a minute is seldom available for its attainment. So short a time allows merely a rough estimate to be formed with the help of the finger.

It is of great importance to the practitioner that this estimate should be in every case as rapid and as accurate as possible; and it behoves the student to acquire experience in this matter at an early period of his clinical training.

The practical method usually recommended has three stages:

(1) *The obliteration of the artery by pressure;*
(2) *The proof that this result has been attained;*
(3) *The estimation of the pressure employed.*

(1) The Obliterating Pressure.

This stage of the method needs but slight description. The hand of the observer occupies nearly the same attitude as in feeling the pulse. But in view of the considerable force which may be required, the distal phalanges do not rest with the flat of their pulp on the artery, but the whole finger is arched. If the reader will refer to Fig. 2, p. 21, he will obtain an idea of the position of hand and fingers best adapted to this special purpose. It is there roughly shown how the middle and annular fingers should *transmit their pressure vertically* to the artery. One, two, or even three fingers may be employed in this manner, but it is well to reserve the index in every case as *the exploring or testing finger*.

Fig. 11, which is taken from Dr. Douglas Powell's diagram, shows the effect of the obliterating pressure on the artery.

Fig. 11.

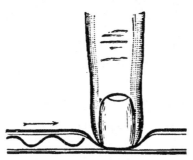

Showing complete stoppage of the pulse by the pressure of the finger.

(2) The Test for Successful Obliteration.

Whenever no pulse can be felt by the index beyond the fingers compressing the artery, we are satisfied that the pressure has told. But, supposing that a beat is still perceived, we must not too readily conclude that obliteration has not taken place. On page 71 will be found a statement of the reasons which suspend our judgment in this matter.

The distal pulse which is felt may be direct or it may be refluent; it may strike the testing finger on its inner side or on its outer side. With the arrangement depicted in Fig. 2, p. 21, it might be supposed that the index finger, which lightly rests on the artery beyond the seat of pressure, would readily perceive the difference. In practice, however, tactile discrimination is exceedingly difficult; and this method is suited only for experienced observers. We must, therefore, urge the beginner to practise at first the following plan :

The Elementary or "Bi-manual" Method of Testing the Nature of the Distal Pulse.*

Remembering that some habitually try the pulse with only one finger, we might assume that a single hand would give a supply of fingers sufficient for any examination. Yet the present method consists in *using both hands to the same pulse.* The object of this lavish manipulation is *first* to ensure that by keeping them separate, the beginner will thoroughly perform the *two functions of applying pressure and of testing the result ;* and *secondly* to enable him more readily to make out whether the wave arises from above or from below, in the manner described on page 71. No difficulty in determining this point can possibly exist when four, or even when three fingers are engaged in testing. Every student should therefore master this easy method before attempting any other.

The "One Hand" Method.

This is the proceeding commonly in use. It has the advantage of greater simplicity and elegance, and leaves one of the hands disengaged. The position of the hand and of the fingers is shown in Fig. 2, p. 21. Pressure is exerted by the middle and annular fingers, which are so bent as to bear vertically on the artery : they are in mutual contact. The index is

---

* The author has pleasure in acknowledging his indebtedness to his senior colleague, Dr. Dickinson, for the suggestion of this method.

placed at a slight distance from them, and is scarcely bent. This finger lies over the artery with the flat of the pulp, not with its tip. The difficult part of this method is how to combine very light pressure of the index with powerful pressure of the other two fingers. Nevertheless, continued practice will enable the observer to perceive even the smallest waves of the pulse.

(3) The Estimation of the Pressure needed for Complete Obliteration of the Pulse.

Having ascertained that the pulse has been obliterated, we proceed with our main object which is to gauge the resisting power of the artery to pressure. In the *bi-manual method* both hands are used with great attention; and whilst the testing hand watches for the disappearance of pulse sensations, the other hand gradually increases its pressure, which had been relaxed for a moment. Meanwhile the amount of energy expended must be estimated by consciousness—in physiological language, *by muscular sense.* The mental estimate thus formed is our measure for the tension of the pulse.

I.

The Pulse of High Arterial Tension.

High blood pressure, whether occurring in a dilated and inelastic, or in a contracted and supple artery, invariably implies *increased cardiac effort.* The greater the resistance in proportion to the heart's strength, so much the longer will be the systoles, and the intervals between them. Therefore not only will the pulse-rate be slow, but the pulse-wave will be less rapid, or of greater length (*pulsus tardus*). *The size of the pulse is in itself no indication of the tension.* A pulse may be small and tense. If it be permanently large and tense hypertrophy certainly exists.

The test for high tension is the long duration of the wave under the finger, and the resistance which it offers to compression.

II.

THE PULSE OF LOW ARTERIAL TENSION.

(A) Abnormally low tension means on the one hand *little vascular resistance;* and this may be due to—

1. The arteries being relatively capacious;
2. The quantity of blood within them relatively small;
3. The vessels unduly yielding.

(B) On the other hand it means *a relatively feeble cardiac systole.*

In Corrigan's pulse (see p. 79) we have an instance of a very low tension, due to the operation of causes 1. 2. and 3. in spite of a very powerful cardiac systole. *In cardiac dilatation* on the contrary, causes 1. 2. and 3. are usually not present, but the cardiac systole is un-equal to the task of keeping up the necessary tension. Just as in *high tension the tendency is towards a slow pulse-rate* and a lingering pulse-wave, *in low tension due to cardiac dilatation rapidity of rate* and shortness of wave are the usual condition. If hypertrophy should co-exist, or should there be any tonic influence, medicinal or otherwise, the pulse-wave and also the pulse-rate may improve. But so long as the heart remains greatly dilated, the occasional occurrence of rather strong beats only serves to accentuate the smallness of others.

III.

THE PULSE IN MITRAL REGURGITATION (NOT COMPLICATED WITH CARDIAC FAILURE).

The features are mainly negative, but so constant in their occurrence as to be diagnostic.

The regurgitant mitral pulse—

is not regular
is not even
is not large
is not strong
is not tense.

Often in the absence of any marked failure of the heart, but invariably when compensation has broken down, the pulse becomes

very irregular
very uneven
very small
very weak
very frequent.

Nevertheless under the use of heart tonics, or when the general health is at its best, intervals occur during which the pulse-rate is moderate, and the pulse may be of tolerable size and regularity.

IV.

THE PULSE IN MITRAL STENOSIS (NOT COMPLICATED WITH HEART FAILURE).

The peculiarities of this pulse are, as might have been surmised, exactly the reverse of those of mitral regurgitation. In one particular, however, the two diseases agree, viz., *in the small size of the beats.* But in mitral stenosis the pulse is

> *relatively infrequent ;*
>
> *regular ;*
>
> *even ;*
>
> *tense ,*
>
> *lingering (pulsus tardus).*

Thus whereas the clinical symptoms and the aspect do not always avail to decide the diagnosis between an onward and a regurgitant murmur, the pulse may afford us a very decisive answer.

V.

The Pulse of Aortic Regurgitation.

Corrigan's Pulse—or Water-hammer Pulse.

This remarkable pulse is commonly called Corrigan's pulse, because it was first described by that celebrated physician.

The water-hammer, after which it is also named, is an instrument in physics, which demonstrates by contrast the uses of the cushion of air normally filling spaces apparently empty. A stout glass tube containing a short column of water is sealed whilst the water is boiling, and allowed to cool. Whenever the tube, thus deprived of its complement of air, is rapidly inverted, the column of water strikes with a sharp shock, resembling the blow of a hammer, the lower end of the tube.

This experiment is very closely imitated by the pulse in cases of *incompetence, i.e.,* imperfect closure, of the aortic valves. The arteries, it is true, are not

rigid like glass, neither do they contain a vacuum such
as we have described, for they immediately contract
whenever their contents diminish.   But in both cases
the fluid is unopposed in its progress by any considerable resistance, and strikes against the finger with a
shock reminding one of the stroke of a hammer.

The Tactile Characters of Corrigan's Pulse.

The features of this pulse, easily recognised by the
finger, are therefore the following :

(a) *collapsed (partly emptied) calibre during the
intervals ;*

(b) *Large, hard and jerky ventricular wave,* the
shock of which, like that of the water-hammer, is
surprisingly sudden and great.

(c) The third feature is no less striking ; it has no
simile elsewhere.   Almost as suddenly as the wave
has appeared, it vanishes again.   The *pulse seems to
pass rapidly from a very large size to almost nothing.*
This early and sudden collapse is typical; and it is
for this sign that the pulse is tested whenever aortic
regurgitation is suspected.

Why the Patient's Hand is to be Elevated in Testing for this Pulse.

In order to intensify the peculiarity just mentioned
the patient's *arm may be held up vertically.*   Thereby
the ventricular wave will hardly lose much of its
strength, but the blood will drain away with increased
rapidity and completeness after the beat.   If any doubt
had been felt as to the existence of aortic reflux, it
would be dispelled by this experiment.

N.B.—*In this disease the arterial blood escapes in both* *directions: onwards* into the capacious capillary system and *backwards* into the ventricle. When the hand is maintained elevated, the second of these outflows would be greatly favoured. The venous blood being also drained away, the hand becomes exsanguine. The normally erect posture of the head would presumably tend towards the same mechanical result. This should be borne in mind in connection with any symptoms of disturbed cerebral circulation arising in cases of regurgitant aortic disease.

The Visible Characters of Corrigan's Pulse.

Very large and sudden wave,—early, complete and sudden subsidence, this is precisely the combination which would lead to visible oscillations in the superficial arteries. And, as a fact, a good observer soon learns to diagnose the sufferers from aortic regurgitation *at first sight,* and merely from the character of their pulsation. The *carotid pulse,* normally visible only in a few subjects, is here *painfully evident.* The carotid being nearer the heart has a larger share than distant arteries, both of the excess of impulse and of the regurgitation. It beats therefore with considerable violence. The same features are visible on a smaller scale in the pulse at the wrist.

The Progress of the Wave (according to Theory).

A priori, what should we expect to take place on the approach of a big wave in a soft, elastic tube which had almost been sucked empty? Precisely that which we observe under similar circumstances in a thin india-rubber tube partly collapsed by atmospheric pressure. Far from opposing any resistance to the penetration of fluid, the elastic walls fly asunder with as much

F

force as was expended in causing their collapse. Whereas in health the advancing wave may have to contend not only with the *weight of so much arterial blood* ahead, but also with some *remaining tension* or *stretch of the arterial wall, with aortic reflux*, presumably, neither of these obstacles would obtain; and the strength of the wave would be propagated to the periphery almost undiminished. This result would be all the more striking since the wave leaving the heart is larger and more abrupt than normal.

The Artery between the Beats (as Observed).

Although we have freely dwelt on the *collapsing character* of the pulse the student should be warned against interpreting these words in too literal a sense. Let him remember that our statements *refer to that which is felt*, not strictly to *that which is*. Having made this reservation we may now refer to another name given to the water-hammer pulse. It has sometimes been termed *the pulse of unfilled arteries*, inasmuch as except for a moment the contents of the arteries are greatly inferior to the maximum arterial capacity. *The name is not a good one;* it mentions imperfect filling which is common to several other conditions, but does not refer to the peculiarities which exclusively belong to this form of pulse. Moreover it allows room for the misconception pointed out above. Let us state once more that arteries are never empty, even in aortic regurgitation. Indeed patients with this disease often enough display to the eye the permanently full state of some of their arteries. The heart, after all, can only accommodate a small quantity of the total arterial contents during its diastole, and in many cases the gap in the valve is too small to allow much back flow. It may be asserted that it is owing to the persistent fulness of arteries even in this affection, that the change about to be described is capable of arising.

Arterial Elongation and Tortuosity.
The Locomotor Pulse.

On close inspection the radial artery is seen to undergo with each beat a powerful and sudden distension. Not only is its calibre visibly increased, almost enabling the eye to follow the progress of the pulse-wave, but the artery also elongates in a noticeable manner. Owing however to the fibrous connections of the arterial sheath, the elongation cannot be linear, like that of a rigid tube, but sooner or later leads to the *formation of broad curves, or of loops.* With each recurring systole these curves undergo *visible displacement.* Hence the name *locomotor pulse* which has been given to this condition.

Tortuosity of an artery, as a permanent change, has already been mentioned among the signs of diminished elasticity. Tortuous pulses are almost always locomotor, because under the powerful wave from the hypertrophied left ventricle, some of the curves tend to be straightened after the fashion of the tubular spring of an aneroid barometer, while other curves are rendered more convex. In both cases, immediately after the passage of the wave, the vessel returns with a jerk to its previous position.

VI.

The Pulse of Aortic Valvular Obstruction.

The difference between this pulse and that of aortic regurgitation is analogous to the differences already described between the two varieties of pulse in mitral disease.

The chief distinguishing features are ·

(1) *Slowness of rate.*

(2) *Laboured and lingering character of wave.*

These are the natural results of the obstacle to the discharge of the ventricular contents, and of the unavoidable prolongation of the ventricular systole.

(3) *A distinct smallness in comparison with the waterhammer pulse.*

(4) *Tension and strength*—because the ventricle hypertrophies under the stimulus of constant effort.

(5) *Evenness.*

(6) *Regularity.*

The remaining features of this pulse are not readily detected by the finger, but can be demonstrated with the sphygmograph.

CHAPTER VI.

ASYNCHRONISM AND INEQUALITY OF THE
PULSES. THE METHODS OF TESTING FOR
EQUALITY OF PULSE-BEATS, AND FOR
IDENTITY OF PULSE-TIME AT THE TWO
WRISTS.

IN the absolutely normal subject the two radial pulses
are synchronous, and of the same size. *Disparity in
size* is of common occurrence and often due to causes
not implying disease, but *want of synchronism* is both
uncommon and of serious import, being usually the
result of *aneurysm*.

I.

HOW TO TEST FOR EQUALITY OF THE TWO RADIAL PULSES.

This inquiry may be sufficiently easy when the
pulses are very different; but it is apt to be exceedingly difficult, if the difference be slight; and opposite
opinions as to which pulse is the larger one are often
given by separate observers, of the same patient.
In this connection it should be mentioned that unequal
pulses often *differ in other respects* as well as in size;
and according as observers are severally struck by one
or by the other difference, so their verdicts may be

various. It is enough however for the beginner to compare the two pulses *as to volume only.*

Delicacy of touch is a special gift with some; with most of us it requires education. The other indispensable requisite is *identity of the experimental conditions.* The two wrists must be in identically similar positions whilst being felt—and the observer must handle the two pulses in some identical fashion.

The two best Positions for the Patient's Hands.

(1) The most favourable attitude is the sitting posture. Both forearms are to rest with their ulnar border on a small table on the other side of which the observer takes his position. The wrists and fingers are gently flexed so as to bring the right and the left knuckles into contact. In this way the two radial arteries are arranged symmetrically and form part of the same semicircular curve. We may term this *the first position.*

(2) In *the second position* the patient is seated, as before. His hands are in front of him; but, instead of being end to end, they overlap, one being slightly in front of the other, as shown in Fig. 12. In this manner the two wrists are in the middle line and separated only by the thickness of the arm

The two Methods which the Observer may adopt.

In both cases the observer is to face the patient.

(1) *If the bimanual method* be used the two pulses are alternately tested, the right with the observer's left hand, and the left pulse with the right hand. The obvious objection to this method is that the two hands may not possess the same delicacy of touch. It is

necessary therefore to check the result first obtained, by crossing the hands so that the right hand feels the right pulse and the left hand is subsequently applied to the left pulse. Should the same difference be again detected between the pulses, it may be assumed to be a real one.

(2) The other method does not entail the same risk of error, and *is far preferable.* It consists in feeling both pulses in succession *with the same hand.* This may be carried out whilst the patient is in either of the two positions described above. If however the second of these positions be adopted, the pulses will be compared with a minimum displacement of the observer's hand. In conclusion we may therefore recommend *the one hand method and the patient's second position as the most perfect combination* for an accurate observation.

II.

How to Test for Synchronism in the Two Pulses.

Here again the same two positions are available for the patient, and one of two methods may be chosen by the observer. The pulses in this case are to be felt simultaneously.

If the bimanual method be preferred, it will matter little how far apart the hands may be kept. The capacity for appreciating minute differences in time between sensations conveyed to the two hands probably varies considerably in individuals.

The majority will probably find it much easier to detect asynchronism with the fingers of *the same hand* than with the two hands separately. We are already trained to this method by the ordinary experience of feeling the pulse with two or three fingers. They

correctly appreciate the feeble interval of time which
elapses between the moments when the first finger and
the last are struck by the wave. I have therefore

Fig. 12.

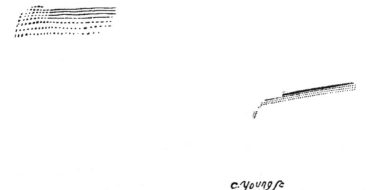

*Easy mode of detecting delay in one of the two pulses. The hands
are sketched as they are seen by the patient.*

been led to adopt the method represented in the
figure.

The patient's hands are to be placed in the second
of the two positions described above, his right wrist
being nearest to his chest, his left wrist immediately in

front of the right, and therefore nearest to the observer. The latter now *grasps both wrists under his right hand*, the left wrist fitting in between the thumb and index, whilst the three remaining fingers reach over the radial border of the right arm. With a little practice the full-grown hand has no difficulty in spanning both wrists. It is important however to manage their fixation entirely by means of the thumb and the annular and little finger. The special office of the index and of the medius is to find the two pulses, and to feel attentively for any difference in time, if it should exist. For the better control of the two wrists (the patient being at first awkward and stiff), it may be advisable to support them and hold them in contact from below with the left hand.

Check Observations Essential.

However great the care bestowed upon the operations described in this chapter, it should be an invariable rule to compare one's own results with those of another observer; and a third opinion, of greater experience, may have to be obtained. Thereby additional confidence will be gained by good observers, whilst others will be made conscious of a need for further practice.

CHAPTER VII.

CAPILLARY PULSATION.

CAPILLARY blood-vessels, even when dilated, are not singly visible to the naked eye. Yet we may judge of their size with some accuracy, thanks to their vast numbers, their close order, and their transparency. The blood, showing through their walls, gives rise to varying effects of colour (*i.e.* complexion) according to its amount.

The larger blood-vessels, on the contrary, having opaque walls, and lying at a greater depth, do not contribute in the same manner to the colouration of surfaces.

Elasticity and Contractility of Capillaries.

Capillaries are in a high degree dilatable and elastic; holding much blood when dilated, they almost exclude blood from their channel when contracted. The result of dilatation is *Flush*, and the result of contraction is *Pallor*. The flush or the pallor may be passing or lasting; if the latter, we infer (excluding of course changes in the quality and quantity of the blood as a whole) that the change in calibre is rather a passive than an active one, and that the capillary dilatation or contraction is in connection with a *local* supply of too much or too little blood.

To what extent true capillaries are *capable of active and independent contraction* long remained a vexed question, all the more difficult to solve owing to the high degree in which the same properties are manifested by arterioles. They are now known to possess a contractility of their own, but it is still admitted that the arterioles are the most active, although not the only, regulators of the blood-supply to the capillary area, and therefore of the calibre of capillaries themselves.

Capillary Pulsation normally Absent.

Since blushing and blanching are visible, any systolic and diastolic variations in the calibre of capillaries should also be visible, especially if occurring on a large scale. No change of this kind is perceptible in health. From this we infer that normally capillaries do not pulsate; and that the pulse-wave is extinguished before it reaches them, by the large frictional and elastic resistances of the arterioles.

Pathological Occurrence of Capillary Pulsation.

In some functional and mechanical defects of the circulation this rule does not apply and capillaries may pulsate. It is then obvious that the peripheral resistances must have diminished, or the force of the systole must have increased beyond the normal; or perhaps that both changes may have occurred together. A full discussion of this subject would take us beyond the elementary lines to which we are bound. It will suffice for the student to remember that relaxation of the arterioles is the main cause of the transmission of a pulse-wave to the capillaries, because it increases the width of the blood channels, and because it removes the buffer-action which arterioles normally oppose to the systolic shock.

THE METHODS FOR DETECTING CAPILLARY PULSATION.

The conditions which render capillary pulsation perceptible generally require to be brought about; they seldom chance to be ready made. The facility with which it may be detected varies much with the natural tint of the complexion, and with the range of the oscillations which occur in the calibre of the capillaries. Under the most favourable circumstances it *is not easily seen at first* by the untrained, and requires to be pointed out to most beginners. Although lying at the surface, it is not an obtrusive phenomenon, and for this reason its existence was probably not even suspected until Quincke called attention to it. An important reason explaining the long delay of this discovery is the fact that those who are the subjects of capillary pulsation are apt to be pallid (as in chlorosis and aortic regurgitation), whilst an essential for the detection of this pulsation is the existence of a *capillary flush of which the variations may be watched.*

The production and the observation of this flush lie at the root of the three methods which have been devised for the clinical demonstration of capillary pulsation. We may conveniently refer to them under the following names,

    I. *The " tache " method.*

    II. *The " lip " method.*

    III. *The " nail " method.*

All three should be tried first in *the healthy subject,* in order to demonstrate the normal absence of this sign;

and next in cases of *extensive aortic regurgitation,* where they will never fail. For the diagnosis of this disease they possess much value.

I. The "Tache" Method.

Leaving aside theoretical questions as to the mechanism of production of the *tache cérébrale* of Trousseau (which he believed to be diagnostic of tubercular meningitis), we will simply deal with the transitory cutaneous blush obtainable in all persons after a sharp and short local stimulation. For our present purpose the abdomen is not the part best suited. We would rather select a situation such as the *forehead,* where the cutaneous capillaries are, under normal circumstances, very active, where the skin is somewhat thin and slightly on the stretch, and especially where it immediately overlies a bony surface.

The tache originally observed by Quincke was brought out by the pressure of a tightly fitting hat. This accidental experiment contains a useful suggestion. Instead of the rough and inelegant proceeding of drawing a finger across the forehead, let a band or belt, or better still a light strap, be tightened round the forehead; a *tache* will then be produced *secundum artem,* and without much, if any, discomfort to the patient.

How to Examine the Tache for Pulsation.

If the patient be pale, any existing capillary pulsation may be sufficiently marked to reveal itself to the first attentive look, the pink patch almost disappearing after each pulsation. More often however the blush is so deep that the pulsatile change in colour is merely a change in the intensity of the red. Even here however more telling *alternations of pallor and of injection will be found at the periphery of the patch*, over a zone of varying width; and it is this region that we should more especially scrutinize. The ability to perceive the capillary pulse is in great measure a matter of visual accommodation. The focal distance for fine perception of colour is not the same as that for clear definition of outline; and therefore we should almost avoid looking at the surface-texture of the skin. From thirty to forty centimetres is the distance usually recommended. Each observer however must find for himself the range at which the colour changes will best strike the eye; and for the same reason he should not neglect to move the head towards and away from the patch under obser vation, before finally concluding that pulsation is not present in it.

II.   The "Lip" Method.

Inasmuch as the patch to be watched is in this case a pale patch, this method is the converse of the preceding; but since in both cases an alternation of pale and of pink is the object sought for, the results will be identical. The patient's lower lip is to be everted; and on its mucous surface is applied with gentle pressure the flat surface of a glass slide. This will produce a central patch of pallor. We now watch through the glass the outer margin of the pale patch; and we shall see there, as we did on the forehead, the alternate coming and going of the pink blush.

There is nothing objectionable or painful in this method, which requires good light and therefore if possible a sitting posture of the patient, facing the window.

III. The "Nail" Method.

This is in principle the same as the lip method. The pale patch has its seat under the nail instead of under the lip. The very gentle pressure required is set up by the tip of the observer's nail applied over the tip of the patient's nail so as to slightly bend the latter. The margin of the blanched patch is to be watched for the pink pulsation as in the preceding experiment.

The " nail to nail " method has this special advantage that the observer can watch simultaneously his own, presumably normal, capillary blush as a standard of comparison. Moreover it is possible to vary and regulate to a nicety the pressure and therefore the depth of the capillary injection. Lastly the experiment can be kept up for any length of time.

BACKWARD OR REGURGITANT CAPILLARY PULSATION.

A capillary pulse may be obtained in cases of extreme tricuspid valvular defect. It was first described by Grocco in 1885. It may be observed under the nail in the same manner as the direct capillary pulse.

Mode of Distinguishing the Backward from the Onward Capillary Pulsation.

In addition to the assistance derived from the existence of a venous pulsation of regurgitant type, two rules are given by Grocco, either of which should enable us to establish the character of the pulsation.

(I) The backward capillary pulse is *not abolished*, as would be the case with the onward pulsation, by compression of the subclavian, of the brachial, or of the radial artery of the same side ;

(2) The pink blush *precedes the radial pulse*, instead of following upon it, as the onward capillary pulsation must do.

LOCAL THROBBING.

Capillary pulsation, if excessive, may show itself by visible change in volume. The variation of colour which was described above implies alternating phases of hyperæmia and of pallor; but should the amount of blood stored in a part be very large, *though pulsation may occur, pallor will not.* Each systole will effect further distension in previously overloaded vessels; and the tissues themselves will be further stretched, in short will pulsate. *Throbbing may be subjective*, that is, it may be felt when it cannot be seen. Usually however the feeling of throbbing corresponds to an active visible throbbing of the part, and of this it would be possible with suitable apparatus to take a tracing. The condition in question may be artificially produced by placing an india-rubber band round the thumb. It is painfully obvious in abscesses, and especially in the variety known as whitlow.

Similar oscillations of volume of slighter extent are continually occurring in our limbs and organs; and in some situations they can be made visible *by the plethysmograph.*

CHAPTER VIII.

VENOUS PULSATION.

————•◆•————

THE subject of this chapter is a large one, ill-suited for exhaustive treatment in these pages. A brief sketch however should be of use to the clinical student; and this will be most conveniently divided into two sections,

    I. *Venous pulsation in general*, the theoretical part, and

    II. *Pulsation in particular veins, and especially in the jugular veins*, the practical and essentially clinical part of the inquiry.

————————

I.

VENOUS PULSATION IN GENERAL.

Setting aside the rhythmic venous pulsations in the bat's wing, originally described by Wharton Hood, and the pulsation of the cardiac extremity of the pulmonary veins in various animals and in man, *veins do not normally pulsate*. Nor is this a matter for wonder, since they are separated from the cardiac influence by the non-pulsatile capillary circulation.

In disturbed function, or as the result of disease,

not only the capillaries (*see* p. 91), but the veins also may present a pulsation.

Venous Pulsation a tergo ; Venous Pulsation a fronte.

Whereas capillaries are usually restricted to a pulsation *a tergo*, the pulsation of veins very commonly arises *a fronte*.   We recognise accordingly two varieties, the *onward venous pulse* and the *backward venous pulse*.

The onward pulse is derived from the *left ventricle* and propagated through the whole circuit as far as the veins.

The backward pulse is due to the systole of the *right ventricle* and often also of the *right auricle*.

Their respective Districts.

Owing chiefly to the obstacle opposed to a venous reflux by the valves of veins, *any pulsation in the smaller peripheral veins is almost invariably onward in character.* For the same reason, and for various others also, the *true pulsation of large, centrally placed veins is invariably backwards.*

True or Direct, and False or Communicated Venous Pulsation.

Before proceeding any further the student must realise that since most veins take their course at no great distance from arteries, *arterial pulsation may be conveyed to them.*   It is essential therefore in every case to determine whether the pulsation is truly venous, or only falsely so called.

In addition to the common form of transmitted

pulsation, we are enabled, with the ophthalmoscope, to witness another variety of venous pulsation communicated, from the arteries, it is true, though not directly (since no pulsation can be seen in them), but through the medium of *pulsatile variations in the intra-ocular pressure.*

In tricuspid incompetence the retinal veins not in frequently pulsate, *as a result of venous reflux.*

How to Tell One from the Other.

This is not always possible, but the attempt should be made. In aspect the transmitted (arterial) pulsation is *more abrupt and shock-like* than the truly venous, which may be recognised by its *soft undulatory movement.* In order to show the spurious character of this pulsation, endeavour by light pressure applied to the artery to isolate it from the vein. Or it may sometimes be possible to abolish the arterial pulsation above the position of the vein under observation and without causing any compression of the latter. Most commonly however the slightest touch, by causing indirect pressure on the vein, interferes with the pulsation.

The Onward Venous Pulsation and its Causes.

True venous pulsation, of onward direction, occurs chiefly, if not exclusively, in the peripheral venules and veins adjoining the capillary distribution. Its occasioning cause is analogous to that which leads to capillary pulsation. The blood channels are so much relaxed as to offer no absolute obstacle to the passage of the pulse-wave; and this is continued, through the capillary district, into the veins as far as a continuous column of blood, unbroken by valves, extends within them.

Complete relaxation of the arterioles and capillaries is often *limited to a special locality, as in inflammation.* Veins under these circumstances may pulsate visibly. The same is true of veins coming from glands in active secretion.   But arterio-capillary relaxation may be *a general process*, and lead to peripheral venous pulsation in many situations.   This may be the result of disease, or it may occur as a temporary and functional change. The effect of a *full meal*, especially combined with *alcoholic stimulation*, will be to quicken the heart's action whilst strengthening it, and at the same time to relax the arterioles *(febris a prandio).*

Whilst this condition lasts, it is sometimes possible to detect pulsation in subcutaneous veins of moderate size, especially at the palms, at the soles, and over the face, forehead, nose, and ears ; these being the situations where, according to Sucquet,* communication normally takes place between arterioles and venules only slightly superior in size to capillaries.

King's Method of Demonstrating Venous Pulsation.

In order the more readily to observe and demonstrate the onward venous pulse King† used fine threads of sealing wax placed across the vein and fastened with wax to the skin close to it, so that any variation in the vein would be indicated by the long end of the thread projecting beyond the vein.   To this arrangement he gave the name of *sphygmoscope.*   This was the *earliest pattern of the lever sphygmograph which is now in use.*

---

* *See* Ozanam, *loc. cit.*, p. 1007.
† *Guy's Hosp. Rep.*, 1837, vol ii. p. 107.

The Backward or Regurgitant Venous Pulse.
Its Causes.

This is the only form of venous pulsation which the
student need study at first. The cause of backward
pulsation is invariably dilatation of the right auricle,
and of the great veins opening into it, by a permanent
overload of blood. The orifice of the venæ cavæ, closing
imperfectly, does not then exclude the blood which they
contain from the influence of the right auricular systole;
if at the same time, as is usually the case, the tricuspid
valve should be incompetent, the right ventricular
systole also takes effect upon the column of venous
blood.

A more detailed consideration of the backward venous
pulse belongs to the second section of this chapter.

II.

Pulsation in Particular Veins.—Pulsation in the Jugulars and their Tributaries.

Its Limits.

The jugulars are the chief site for visible true backward venous pulse; and this is readily seen, though not
easily told, from the transmitted arterial pulsation which
is so commonly present in them. The regurgitant
venous pulse commonly extends into the facial vein
and its tributaries, and sometimes into the *brachial*.
The extension of the pulsation is limited according to
the length of the continuous column of blood filling the
veins; where this stops, there also stops the pulsation. If the vein be full from end to end, the pulse

will not always be propagated through the whole column, but may only affect part of it.

Marey is stated to have once observed reflex venous pulsation in varicose veins of the leg* in a subject affected with disease of the right side of the heart. It is very rare, however, to trace the reflex venous pulse through the inferior vena cava beyond the hepatic veins, or through the superior vena cava beyond the brachial veins.

Backward Jugular Pulsation and Backward Jugular Flow (or Regurgitation).

These two conditions are often associated, but not of necessity. It is easily conceivable and probably often occurs that, *without any reflux*, venous pulsation should be transmitted through the thin jugular valves stretched across an otherwise continuous column of blood which has been simply retarded in its onward progress by an over full condition of the right side of the heart. This condition is quite different from the graver defect in which not only a pulse-wave, but a flow of blood finds its way into the vein. *Regurgitation of the blood from the auricle* into the jugulars may be taken as a proof that not only the tricuspid valve, but also the jugular valve is incompetent; and, whenever reflux takes place, jugular pulsation is necessarily present also.

METHODS FOR ASCERTAINING THE PRESENCE OF REFLUX INTO THE JUGULAR VEIN.

The presence or the absence of regurgitation from the heart may generally be made clear with the help

---

* Ozanam, *loc. cit.*, p. 1007.

of a simple experiment. The contents of the distended jugulars are pushed away *by running the finger in an upward direction along the vessel.* If the tricuspid valves be incompetent a fresh quantity of blood may be sent into the emptied channel by the next ventricular systole. Should they be competent, no reflux will take place.

The Subcostal Pressure Method.

Another method is based upon a mode of exploration suggested by Dr. Pasteur " for the purpose of estimating the condition of the right side of the heart."[*] " Under certain circumstances, a distension or overfilling of the external jugular veins, apparently from below, with or without pulsation or undulation, takes place when pressure is exerted in the right hypochondriac or epigastric regions with the flat of the hand, the direction of pressure being backwards and upwards." As a result of a procedure of this kind, if the jugular valve be incompetent, a regurgitation would be occasioned into the jugular through the intermediary of the inferior vena cava, of the right auricle, and of the superior vena cava, all of which are supposed to be distended with blood. In looking for this sign the observer should remember that he is dealing with a congested and extremely tender organ.

THE PRÆSYSTOLIC AND THE SYSTOLIC JUGULAR PULSATIONS.

Let us now examine more closely the backward venous pulsation noticeable at the root of the neck in cases of tricuspid and jugular incompetence. As

---

[*] *The Lancet*, May 15, 1886.

regards time this form of pulsation is *always either systolic or præsystolic (auricular-systolic)*.

A diastolic retraction of the jugular during each cardiac diastole has been described among the signs of pericardial adhesions ; but this diastolic negative pulse has nothing to do with the valvular affections we are now considering. Since neither the superior nor the inferior vena cava possess any valves capable of periodically closing their cardiac orifice, reflux into them with each auricular systole might have been regarded as normal and unavoidable. This is however pre vented by the *fine adjustment* of the auricular fibres surrounding the orifices ; and by the fact that the blood is urged onward into the ventricle as *in the direction of least resistance*. Both these arrangements are disturbed *when the auricular wall is stretched* by the presence of *too large* a quantity of blood, and when the passage of blood into the ventricle becomes difficult. As we might expect, the overloaded auricle then sets up a backward pulsation in the jugular at the moment of its own contraction, that is, immediately before the ventricular systole.

This auricular or præsystolic pulsation is known by its time, by its rapidity and short duration, and frequently also by the double oscillation of which it is composed.

Upon this usually follows the *systolic or ventricular pulse-wave*, known by its larger size and greater duration. Very often this wave alone is perceptible.

Varying Degree of Jugular Distension as Affecting the Pulsation.

In addition to the pulsations just described, further changes are connected with the varying degree of distension of the veins, under the influence of lessening or increasing impediments to the circulation. In the foregoing description we have imagined the jugulars to be kept permanently full. But matters are often complicated by *their fulness not being constant but intermittent;* and, therefore, the visible pulsation being also intermittent. It then becomes necessary to distinguish between a *true blood reflux* and a mere *refluent blood-wave.*

Inspection of the Episternal Notch and of the Supra-clavicular Fossæ.

A mere inspection of these regions affords valuable indications. The student will note the absence—

(1) *Of venous fulness,*

(2) *Of transmitted arterial pulsation,*

(3) *Of true venous pulsation:*

or if these be present he will proceed to describe them. In addition to inspection, palpation (*especially deep palpation*) of the *episternal notch and of the supra-clavicular fossæ* will help us in determining whether a jugular pulsation may be merely the arterial beat communicated from the arch of *the aorta and from the innominate* (a frequent occurrence); or, as in the case of the subclavian venous pulsation, one propagated from the *subclavian artery.*

Backward Pulsation into the Inferior Vena Cava. Hepatic Pulsation, Spurious and True.

The over full condition of the right auricle must make itself felt, not only in the superior vena cava and the jugulars, but also in the inferior vena cava. Into this vein *the capacious hepatic veins* open just below the diaphragm, and they receive a share of the regurgitated wave.

Commonly, however, the pulsation is limited to the primary divisions of these large veins The liver itself, already subjected to passive pulsation by contact with the distended right heart, receives an additional impulse from the regurgitation into the hepatic venous trunks. The resulting movements of the organ may properly be designated as *transmitted*.

In a few cases the intra-hepatic circulation is more deeply influenced, and the regurgitant pulsation, extending down the hepatic venous system, produces at each systole a *perceptible increase in the volume of the liver.* If this organ, which, under these circumstances, is always enlarged, be palpated as closely as possible between the two hands, *a distensile pulse* will be perceived at each systole. *This is true pulsation of the liver*, as opposed to the *transmitted, spurious,* hepatic pulsation, or common *diffused hepatic impulse*, described in the preceding paragraph.

Arterial Hepatic Pulsation.

It will be noticed that the *true hepatic pulse is usually regarded as a venous and a regurgitant one.* Since however both the hepatic artery and the hepatic vein are continuous with the portal capillaries, pulsation might conceivably be propagated to the latter *from the hepatic artery.* This would be *a direct or arterial hepatic pulsation.* Conceivably also pulsation might arise in one and the same case from both artery and vein. As regards time, a slight difference would exist between the longer circuit of the direct arterial pulsation from the left ventricle, and the shorter route taken by the refluent pulsation from the right auricle.

Theoretically a single impulse would be proof that the hepatic pulsation was entirely of one kind. But in practice, since the delay between the venous and the arterial wave is trifling, it would be exceedingly difficult to decide, on this ground alone, and in the absence of the usual signs of dilatation of the right auricle and ventricle, whether the pulsation was venous or arterial.

GLOSSARY OF TERMS

IN USE AT THE PRESENT TIME OR IN THE PAST, IN CONNECTION WITH THE PULSE.*

—+♦+—

Abdominal pulsation
Abortive beats
Accessory beats
Allorhythmia (see p. 63)
Anacrotic pulse
Anacrotism (secondary wave during the ascent)
Anastomosis
Ant-like pulse (faintest pulsation)
Aortic pulse
Arhythmia or *Arrhythmia* (see p. 64
Asynchronism
Auricular pulsation

Bigeminal pulse
Bounding pulse

Capillary pulsation
Cerebral pulsation
Collapsing pulse
Compressible pulse
Corrigan's pulse

Dicrotic or dicrotous pulse
Dicrotism (secondary beat or wave in the pulse)

Diffluent pulse
Direct pulse
Distal pulse

Epigastric pulsation
Equal pulse
Even pulse
Eurhythmia (normal rhythm)

Faint pulse
Faltering pulse
Flabby pulse
Flagging pulse
Fœtal pulse
Frail pulse
Frequent pulse
Full pulse

Hard pulse
Hectic pulse
Hepatic pulsation
Heterochronism
Heteromorphism
High tension of pulse
Hurried pulse
Hyperdicrotism (excessive dicrotism)

---

* For an explanation of the few English words of which the meaning is not obvious, the reader is referred to the corresponding page.

Many obsolete expressions have been left out which would not be understood without an account of the erroneous pulse-theories upon which they were based.

Ictus (the actual beat)
Incompressible pulse (see p. 67)
Inequality
Infrequent pulse
Intermittent pulse
Irregular pulse

Jerky pulse
Jugular pulse

Katacrotism (secondary wave during the descent)

Laboured pulse
Lean pulse
Linked beats (see p. 6)
Locomotor pulse (see p. 83)
Low tension of pulse (see p. 77)

Meagre pulse
Moderate pulse

Paradoxical pulse (see p. 66)
Pararhythmia (abnormal rhythm)
Peripheral pulse
Poor pulse
Pulsation by anastomosis
Pulse of aneurysm
Pulse of "unfilled arteries"
Pulsus acceleratus, &c. (See Latin list)

Quick pulse

Recurrent pulse
Refluent pulse
Reflux pulse
Regularity of pulse
Regurgitation
Reptation of pulse
Renal pulse
Retardation of pulse
Rhythm

Running pulse

Serpiginous pulse
Senile pulse
Shabby pulse
Shallow pulse
Slender pulse
Slight pulse
Slow pulse
Spurious pulse
Strong pulse
Swift pulse
Stumbling pulse
Symmetrical pulses
Synchronous pulses

Tall pulse
Tense pulse
Thin pulse
Thready pulse
Thrilling pulse
Thumping pulse
Tortuous pulse
Tremulous pulse
Tripping pulse
Trigeminal pulse
Tumbling pulse
Turgid pulse

Vehement pulse
Venous pulse
Ventricular pulse
Vermicular pulse
Vibratory pulse

Uneven pulse

Water-hammer pulse
Wavy pulse
Waxing and waning pulse
Weak pulse
Wiry pulse
Worm-like pulse

LATIN LIST.

Pulsus acceleratus, quickened
   acutus, sharp
   æqualis, even
   alternans (see p. 60)
   altus, deep
   amplus, wide
   angustus, narrow
   apertus, plain ; not latent
   bigeminus (see pp. 60–65)
   bis feriens, dicrotic
   brevis, short
   caprizans, hyperdicrotic
   celer, swift
   citatus, quickened
   concisus, short and defined
   contractus, small
   creber, frequent
   debilis, weak
   deficiens, failing
   differens, unlike its fellow
   difficilis, laboured
   durus, hard
   exilis, thin
   filiformis, thready
   formicans, ant-like
   fortis, strong
   gracilis, slender
   humilis, low, shallow
   impar citatus, irregular
   impetuosus, violent
   inæqualis, uneven

Pulsus inæqualiter inæqualis (see
   p. 60)
   inciduus, waxing and waning
   inordinatus, irregular
   intermittens, intermittent
   intermittens cum inspiratione
   (see p. 66)
   intercidens, interrupted
   intercurrens, with accessory
   beats
   languidus, languid
   latens, latent
   latus, broad
   longus, long
   magnus, large
   manifestus, not latent
   medius, middle-sized
   moderatus, moderate
   mollis, soft
   myurus, like a rat's tail
   obscurus, ill defined
   obtusus, thick
   oppressus, depressed
   ordinatus, regular
   oscillans, oscillating
   paradoxus (see p. 66)
   parvus, small
   plenus, full
   profundus, deep
   rarus, infrequent
   recurrens, recurrent

Pulsus reptans, crawling
    robustus, strong
    serratus, saw-like
    spasticus, jerky
    tardus, slow
    tensus, tense
    tremulus, tremulous
    trigeminus (see pp. 60, 65)

Pulsus turgidus, distended
    undosus, wavy
    vacuus, empty
    validus, strong
    vehemens, vehement
    velox, rapid, swift
    vermicularis, worm-like
    vibratus, vibratile

PRINTED BY BALLANTYNE, HANSON AND CO.
LONDON AND EDINBURGH

CPSIA information can be obtained
at www.ICGtesting.com
Printed in the USA
LVOW04s1629091115

461714LV00022B/1119/P